MOTIVATIONAL INTERVIEWING AND CBT

Applications of Motivational Interviewing
Stephen Rollnick, William R. Miller,
and Theresa B. Moyers, Series Editors
www.guilford.com/AMI

Since the publication of Miller and Rollnick's classic *Motivational Interviewing*, now in its third edition, MI has been widely adopted as a tool for facilitating change. This highly practical series includes general MI resources as well as books on specific clinical contexts, problems, and populations. Each volume presents powerful MI strategies that are grounded in research and illustrated with concrete, "how-to-do-it" examples.

Motivational Interviewing in Health Care:
Helping Patients Change Behavior
Stephen Rollnick, William R. Miller, and Christopher C. Butler

Motivational Interviewing with Adolescents and Young Adults
Sylvie Naar and Mariann Suarez

Motivational Interviewing in Social Work Practice
Melinda Hohman

Motivational Interviewing in the Treatment of Anxiety
Henny A. Westra

Motivational Interviewing, Third Edition: Helping People Change
William R. Miller and Stephen Rollnick

Motivational Interviewing in Groups
Christopher C. Wagner and Karen S. Ingersoll, with Contributors

Motivational Interviewing in the Treatment
of Psychological Problems, Second Edition
Hal Arkowitz, William R. Miller, and Stephen Rollnick, Editors

Motivational Interviewing in Diabetes Care
Marc P. Steinberg and William R. Miller

Motivational Interviewing in Nutrition and Fitness
Dawn Clifford and Laura Curtis

Motivational Interviewing in Schools:
Conversations to Improve Behavior and Learning
Stephen Rollnick, Sebastian G. Kaplan, and Richard Rutschman

Motivational Interviewing with Offenders:
Engagement, Rehabilitation, and Reentry
Jill D. Stinson and Michael D. Clark

Motivational Interviewing and CBT:
Combining Strategies for Maximum Effectiveness
Sylvie Naar and Steven A. Safren

Building Motivational Interviewing Skills, Second Edition:
A Practitioner Workbook
David B. Rosengren

Motivational Interviewing and CBT

Combining Strategies for Maximum Effectiveness

Sylvie Naar
Steven A. Safren

Foreword by William R. Miller

THE GUILFORD PRESS
New York   London

Library of Congress Cataloging-in-Publication Data
Names: Naar-King, Sylvie, author. | Safren, Steven A., author.
Title: Motivational interviewing and CBT : combining strategies for maximum
    effectiveness / Sylvie Naar, Steven A. Safren ; foreword by William R.
    Miller.
Description: NewYork, NY : Guilford Press, [2017] | Series: Applications of
    motivational interviewing | Includes bibliographical references and index.
Identifiers: LCCN 2017017708 | ISBN 9781462531547 (hardcover : alk. paper)
Subjects: LCSH: Motivational interviewing. | Cognitive therapy. |
    Psychotherapy.
Classification: LCC BF637.I5 N2927 2017 | DDC 158.3—dc23
LC record available at *https://lccn.loc.gov/2017017708*

About the Authors

Sylvie Naar, PhD, is Professor and Director of the Division of Behavioral Sciences in the Department of Family Medicine and Public Health Sciences at Wayne State University. She conducts research on the use of MI and MI integrated with CBT to improve health behaviors for many populations. She also studies how best to teach MI and how to implement the approach within organizations. With over 100 publications, Dr. Naar is coauthor of *Motivational Interviewing with Adolescents and Young Adults.* She is a member of the Motivational Interviewing Network of Trainers (MINT) and has provided training locally, nationally, and internationally.

Steven A. Safren, PhD, ABPP, is Professor of Psychology at the University of Miami. Previously, he was Professor of Psychology in Psychiatry at Harvard Medical School and Director of Behavioral Medicine at Massachusetts General Hospital (MGH). He is a past editor of *Cognitive and Behavioral Practice* and an associate editor of the *Journal of Consulting and Clinical Psychology.* Dr. Safren is a recipient of the Pioneer Award for Outstanding Contributions to HIV Adherence Science/Practice from the International Association of Providers of AIDS Care, as well as mentoring/training awards from Division 44 (Society for the Psychological Study of Lesbian, Gay, Bisexual, and Transgender Issues) of the American Psychological Association, Harvard Medical School, and the Division of Psychology Training at MGH. His research and more than 260 publications focus on health-related behavioral interventions and adult attention-deficit/hyperactivity disorder.

Foreword

On first take it might seem that motivational interviewing (MI) and cognitive-behaviorial therapy (CBT) are conceptual opposites. CBT is often practiced from a directive expert model—that as the therapist I have what the client lacks (skills, knowledge, rational thinking) and my job is to install it. "I have what you need, and I will give it to you." MI, in contrast, is not about installing things. It is a way of calling forth (*educare*) that which is already there: the person's own motivations, insight, wisdom, and ideas. What could be more opposite?

Yet it is clear to me that MI and CBT are not only compatible but complementary. My predoctoral training in clinical psychology was at the University of Oregon, where we "Oregon products" were intended to be evidence-based behavior therapists. Yet in our second year of training there was a required year-long practicum on how to work with clients, and by happy coincidence none of the behavioral faculty wanted to teach it that year. So they called in a counseling psychology faculty member who spent the year teaching us the person-centered method and perspectives of Carl Rogers before we got into the actual practice of behavior therapy (Gilmore, 1973).

The next year I was struggling to learn how to do behavioral family therapy, working with parents under the tutelage of a faculty member who had been trained by Gerald Patterson, a pioneering grandfather of social learning methods in parenting (Patterson, 1975). We were teaching parents how to count and track behaviors on gold star charts, with heavy emphasis on positive reinforcement (Miller & Danaher, 1976). It was all very logical, with highly structured homework assignments. The problem, as behavior therapists quickly discover, is that people often do not complete their assignments. It was slow going.

Then we took a field trip over to the Oregon Research Institute to watch Patterson work with a family. As we sat behind the one-way mirror, it struck me that he was doing many things with the family that he had not described in his prolific research and how-to writings. He was warm, engaging, funny, and personable, and he listened carefully to what both parents and children said. You might do *anything* for this fellow (he was that good with interpersonal skills), and I thought, "Oh, *that's* how you do it!" I went back to the psychology clinic and started using those listening skills that I had learned, and the behavior therapy began to work for me. Jerry Patterson himself later became very interested in resistance and the principles of interpersonal influence in behavior therapy and contributed groundbreaking research on the topic (Patterson & Forgatch, 1985; Patterson & Chamberlain, 1994).

Over the years I developed a way of doing behavior therapy in a person-centered style. They just seemed to fit together for me. When I began teaching in the PhD program at the University of New Mexico, I trained students in both behavior therapy and a Rogerian style. Would it matter how skillfully counselors listened to their clients while delivering a manual-guided behavior therapy? During one clinical trial with problem drinkers, we randomly assigned clients to nine different therapists, observing their work via one-way mirrors. Clients of the most empathic therapists were far more successful in reducing their alcohol use than those working with low-empathy therapists. At 6 months we could account for *two-thirds* of the variance in client drinking from the empathic skill level of therapists delivering (allegedly) the very same behavior therapy (Miller, Taylor, & West, 1980), an effect that was still present at 2-year follow-up (Miller & Baca, 1983). The next year Steve Valle (1981) published similar findings: that relapse rates across 2 years of follow-up were two to four times higher for clients working with counselors low in person-centered skills, compared with clients in the same program fortunate enough to get counselors with high interpersonal functioning.

When a group of Norwegian psychologists asked me to demonstrate how I worked with people with alcohol problems, I naturally used a combination of Rogerian and CBT methods. It was out of these discussions that MI was conceived (Miller, 1983). When I first described it I was thinking of MI as a prelude to treatment, something you could do before beginning CBT to "prime the pump" (Miller, 1983). What we quickly found, much to our surprise, was that with a brief MI intervention people often initiated behavior change without further treatment. Subsequently we have continued to explore ways in which mainstream, manual-guided CBT can be delivered and integrated with an MI style (Longabaugh, Zweben, LoCastro, & Miller, 2005; Meyers & Smith, 1995).

With this book, the integration of MI and CBT takes a leap forward. Behavior therapists have, I believe, paid far too little attention to the substantial impact of interpersonal skills and the therapeutic relationship in shaping treatment engagement, retention, adherence, and outcome. One result is the raging debate about the relative importance of "evidence-based" versus "common" factors in psycho-therapy (e.g., Norcross, 2011). Person-centered advocates could, in turn, be faulted for paying too little attention to empirical science in recent decades, though it was Carl Rogers himself who pioneered both process and outcome research in psychotherapy. From an MI perspective, this is clearly a both/and issue (Miller & Moyers, 2015). An evidence-based treatment cannot be separated from the person who delivers it, any more than a race car from its driver or a chef from the quality of a meal. Allegedly "common" factors that influence outcome, such as therapist empathy (Truax & Carkhuff, 1967), may not be all that common in actual prac-tice, and if we call them "nonspecific" it simply means that we have not done our homework. It is time—far past time—to specify, measure, study, and teach inter-personal factors that can have such a large impact on client outcomes.

Perhaps MI and CBT are like oil and water. My junior chemistry project in high school was a study of emulsifying agents that make it possible to blend oil and water. It was a portent of things to come. This book is an emulsifier.

WILLIAM R. MILLER, PhD
Emeritus Distinguished Professor of Psychology and Psychiatry
The University of New Mexico

References

Gilmore, S. K. (1973). *The counselor-in-training*. Englewood Cliffs, NJ: Prentice-Hall.

Longabaugh, R., Zweben, A., LoCastro, J. S., & Miller, W. R. (2005). Origins, issues and options in the development of the combined behavioral intervention. *Journal of Studies on Alcohol (Supplement), 15*, 179–187.

Meyers, R. J., & Smith, J. E. (1995). *Clinical guide to alcohol treatment: The community reinforcement approach*. New York: Guilford Press.

Miller, W. R. (1983). Motivational interviewing with problem drinkers. *Behavioural Psychotherapy, 11*, 147–172.

Miller, W. R., & Baca, L. M. (1983). Two-year follow-up of bibliotherapy and therapist-directed controlled drinking training for problem drinkers. *Behavior Therapy, 14*, 441–448.

Miller, W. R., & Danaher, B. G. (1976). Maintenance in parent training. In J. D. Krumboltz & C. E. Thoresen (Eds.), *Counseling methods* (pp. 434–444). New York: Holt, Rinehart & Winston.

Miller, W. R., & Moyers, T. B. (2015). The forest and the trees: Relational and specific factors in addiction treatment. *Addiction, 110*, 401–413.

Miller, W. R., Taylor, C. A., & West, J. C. (1980). Focused versus broad spectrum behavior therapy for problem drinkers. *Journal of Consulting and Clinical Psychology, 48*, 590–601.

Norcross, J. C. (Ed.). (2011). *Psychotherapy relationships that work: Evidence-based responsiveness* (2nd ed.). New York: Oxford University Press.

Patterson, G. R. (1975). *Families: Applications of social learning to family life* (rev. ed.). Champaign, IL: Research Press.

Patterson, G. R., & Chamberlain, P. (1994). A functional analysis of resistance during patient training therapy. *Clinical Psychology: Science and Practice, 1,* 53–70.

Patterson, G. R., & Forgatch, M. S. (1985). Therapist behavior as a determinant for client noncompliance: A paradox for the behavior modifier. *Journal of Consulting and Clinical Psychology, 53,* 846–851.

Truax, C. B., & Carkhuff, R. R. (1967). *Toward effective counseling and psychotherapy.* Chicago: Aldine.

Valle, S. K. (1981). Interpersonal functioning of alcoholism counselors and treatment outcome. *Journal of Studies on Alcohol, 42,* 783–790.

Acknowledgments

We are grateful to all who helped support the conceptualization, writing, and production of this book, which we hope will be a useful resource for health care and mental health care professionals and our clients. The first thank you goes to Jeffrey Parsons of Hunter College, who introduced us to each other, starting a stimulating and wonderful working relationship and friendship. The staff at The Guilford Press, in general, and Jim Nageotte, in particular, have been a tremendous support throughout the process, providing insight on the direction of the book and helping shape many aspects of the work to be as user-friendly as possible. Special thanks to Lisa Todd for helping prepare the activities. William (Bill) Miller and Steven Rollnick encouraged us to take on the project in the first place, and Bill has been an excellent series editor and helpful resource throughout the process, in terms of providing input on ideas, reviewing chapters for content and flow, and keeping us solidly grounded in the overarching MI framework.

From Sylvie Naar

To Maurice, who showed me the power of change.

To Linda Greer Clark, who helped me experience CBT as I was writing the book.

To my children, Leah and Alex, who are always by my side as I navigate work–life balance.

To my family, who believe I can do anything.

To my research participants, who taught me everything this book has to offer.

Finally, I would like to thank Steve Safren, who did not hesitate to jump right in despite multiple commitments and life changes, and has been a rock throughout this process.

From Steven A. Safren

In addition to those thanked above, I have to acknowledge my husband, William Pirl, for all of his support of me and my career. This book and many others aspects of my career would not have been possible without him. I would also like to mention our two sons, Jared Safren and Seth Safren, who help me see the world from a different perspective every day and whom I love deeply. (I think they will get a kick out of seeing their names published in this book! Hi, Jared! Hi, Seth!) I am also continually inspired by my current and past mentees, who make my job and career so joyful and gratifying. My professional mentors have each had an incredible impact on me in different ways at different times in my development, including, but not limited to, Richard Heimberg, Michael Otto, and Kenneth Mayer. Finally, and most relevant to the current work, I want to thank Sylvie Naar for inviting me to join her on this project, and from whom I have learned an incredible amount about MI and changing health-related behavior. Working with her on this book has truly shaped how I now think about behavioral change interventions, impacting my current and future clinical research projects and how I approach supervising my trainees in addressing complex psychological and behavioral health issues. Thank you so much, Sylvie!

Contents

CHAPTER 1

Integrating Motivational Interviewing and Cognitive-Behavioral Therapy

RATIONALE, APPROACH, AND EVIDENCE

Over the last decade, the field of behavior change has encouraged the integration of different forms of evidence-based treatments by identifying their general factors and shared elements and applying them across multiple behaviors (Abraham & Michie, 2008; Chorpita, Becker, Daleiden, & Hamilton, 2007; Fixsen, Naoom, Blase, Friedman, & Wallace, 2005). General factors, sometimes called "common factors," refer to the personal, interpersonal, and other processes that are shared among all psychosocial treatments—for example, therapeutic alliance, empathy, and optimism. These account for much of treatment outcome beyond the specific treatment techniques. "Shared elements" refer to the components of evidence-based clinical practice that are common across distinct treatment protocols—for example, self-monitoring, cognitive restructuring, and refusal skills (Barth et al., 2012).

Scientists have recently advocated for the study of processes that cut across diseases, a paradigm that fits nicely with the shared elements and factors approach to treatment (Bickel & Mueller, 2009; Norton, 2012). By identifying shared elements and relational factors and applying them across different behaviors and symptoms (with specific adaptation for symptom clusters as necessary), we can promote more widespread dissemination of evidence-based treatments and improve the ease of implementation and training. This approach can more easily address common comorbidities and address multiple behavior change. "Transdiagnostic" or "unified" treatments are defined as those that apply the same underlying treatment principles across conditions or behaviors instead of delivering different specific treatments for different conditions (McEvoy, Nathan, & Norton, 2009). Instead, the protocols are individualized in the treatment planning process. The term "unified" has also been used to refer to unified treatment plans that address mental and physical health such as depression and medication adherence or obesity and substance use. We believe the integration of motivational interviewing (MI) and cognitive-behavioral therapy (CBT) can serve as a unified treatment approach to improve mental and physical health, and we have written this book accordingly.

> By identifying shared elements and relational factors and applying them across different behaviors and symptoms, we can improve implementation and address common comorbidities.

So Why MI?

MI is a collaborative, guiding conversational style used for strengthening a person's own (intrinsic) motivation and commitment for change. After over 30 years of empirical study, MI has proved to be a frontline, evidence-based, successful intervention approach for facilitating positive behavior change, and is increasingly utilized in the areas of substance abuse, mental health, and primary and specialty health care. MI specifies communication behaviors that underlie the relational factors of psychotherapy and thus provides a foundation for client–practitioner communication in multiple settings.

Why CBT?

CBT focuses on changing maladaptive thoughts and behaviors that maintain symptoms and interfere with functioning (Beck, 2011). CBT approaches are some of the most widely disseminated evidence-based treatment elements and they share elements across many diagnoses such as depression, anxiety, substance abuse, attention-deficit/hyperactivity disorder (ADHD), and obesity (Tolin, 2010). CBT is hard work for clients! It requires in-session practice and between-session "homework," work that involves making changes in areas that have been difficult for clients to master in the past. This is why experts (Driessen & Hollon, 2011) say that MI can make CBT work better by specifying strategies to build clients' own motivation to do the hard work, and thereby to help you, as the therapist, avoid being the "bad guy" in this process.

Although CBT has some of the strongest evidence for change in its favor (Hofmann, Asnaani, Vonk, Sawyer, & Fang, 2012), it is also true that many individuals do not respond to treatment, do not adhere to treatment tasks, discontinue treatment prematurely, or, after initial success, are unable to maintain change (LeBeau, Davies, Culver, & Craske, 2013; Naar-King, Earnshaw, & Breckon,

2013). Experts in both CBT and MI have suggested this may be at least in part because some CBT approaches do not specify the skills necessary to support the practitioner's relationship with the client and do not help practitioners strengthen motivation for change at both the onset and during the course of CBT (Driessen & Hollon, 2011; Miller & Moyers, 2015). Thus, integrating MI with CBT may improve both initial response rates and maintenance of change after treatment is completed. MI can make CBT work better!

MI–CBT Integration

MI was originally developed to build motivation for *initial* change; MI strategies for enacting and maintaining change have only recently begun to be specified (Miller & Rollnick, 2012). Miller and Rollnick (2002) note that once initial motivation for change has been established, it may be time to move to more action-oriented treatments such as CBT. Thus, incorporating more action-oriented treatments may strengthen the behavior changes that MI has helped to initiate. Yet motivation still fluctuates in strength and direction during enactment and maintenance of change, suggesting that integrating MI with CBT may create a more potent behavioral treatment than either set of strategies alone.

Westra and Arkowitz (2011) discuss several ways in which MI can be combined with CBT. First, MI may be delivered as a brief pretreatment to build motivation for multisession intervention. Second, MI can be used at specific moments during CBT when client discord or ambivalence arises. Third, MI can serve as an integrative framework in which other interventions, such as CBT strategies, could be delivered. This book addresses all three approaches using concepts from Miller and Rollnick (2012) that can be applied to different behaviors and concerns. As such, the book can be utilized as the beginning of a transdiagnostic protocol to address various processes of change with both MI and CBT as the underlying core. This book is based on the growing body of research and clinical applications of MI integrated with cognitive-behavioral approaches (including our own ongoing work), and it outlines the clinical skills necessary to deliver this integrated treatment.

> Integrating MI with CBT may create a more potent behavioral treatment than either set of strategies alone.

We also attempt to delineate where MI–CBT integration is feasible and readily applicable, and where there may be conflicts between the approaches (see Figure 1.1). Moyers and Houck (2011), commenting on one of the only trials using MI as an integrative framework to deliver CBT (Anton et al., 2006), note that MI and CBT are not always a perfect marriage. There are times when the approaches contradict each other and the practitioner must choose which approach will prevail. In these cases, this book will not attempt to choose a side but rather will illustrate

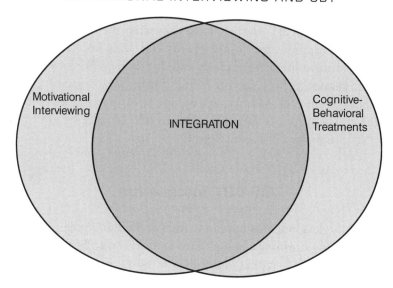

FIGURE 1.1. MI–CBT integration.

your options as discussed in the "MI–CBT Dilemmas" sections at the ends of Chapters 2–8.

What's the Evidence?

Many studies suggest that combining MI with CBT is more effective than usual care in many areas of behavior change such as anxiety (Westra, Arkowitz, & Dozois, 2009), depression with and without comorbid substance use (Riper et al., 2014), cocaine use (McKee et al., 2007); marijuana use (Babor, 2004), smoking cessation (Heckman, Egleston, & Hofmann, 2010), medication adherence (Spoelstra, Schueller, Hilton, & Ridenour, 2015), and weight-related behaviors (Naar-King et al., 2016); however, much less is known about whether either treatment is more effective than a combined treatment approach. The few studies of MI plus CBT compared to MI alone have all targeted substance use and suggest that the combined treatment is often, but not always, more effective than MI alone (Moyers & Houck, 2011). In one meta-analysis (Hettema, Steele, & Miller, 2005), the effect of MI was stronger and lasted longer when combined with another active treatment than when used by itself. Some published trials compared a few sessions of MI as a pretreatment to CBT with CBT alone and found that adding MI improved outcomes for alcohol consumption (Connors, Walitzer, & Dermen, 2002), cocaine use (Stotts, Schmitz, Rhoades, & Grabowski, 2001), generalized anxiety disorder (Westra et al., 2009; Westra & Dozois, 2006), and child behavior problems (Nock

& Kazdin, 2005). To date there are no studies that have compared CBT alone with an integrated MI and CBT approach (i.e., where MI is not just a pretreatment but is integrated throughout treatment). However, two qualitative studies showed that high-empathy counselors were more effective than low-empathy counselors when both provided behavior therapy for alcohol use (Miller, Taylor, & West, 1980; Valle, 1981). In a more recent qualitative study comparing client's perceptions of CBT therapists with more positive and less positive outcomes, clients experienced CBT therapists with more positive outcomes as being more evocative and collaborative, engaging client's expertise, and having more active participation in the treatment process (Kertes, Westra, & Aviram, 2009). As you will see below, these therapists were demonstrating the MI spirit.

To date, studies of transdiagnostic or unified treatments have typically focused on emotional disorders such as the different anxiety diagnoses and depression, often CBT-based with MI as a pretreatment to increase engagement (Folkman, 2011). A review of such studies (McEvoy et al., 2009) suggested that unified treatments are associated with symptom improvement compared to wait-list controls. The unified treatments reviewed typically included CBT elements such as psychoeducation, cognitive restructuring, coping skills, exposure, relaxation training, and behavioral activation. Unified treatments appeared to have similar effect sizes as diagnosis-specific treatments, and there was some evidence to suggest that unified treatments targeting one set of concerns had positive impacts on comorbid conditions or other areas of behavior change. At the time of the McEvoy et al. (2009) review, there were no studies directly comparing a unified treatment to diagnosis-specific treatments. However, a more recent study (Norton, 2012) compared a transdiagnostic group CBT for anxiety disorders (including psychoeducation, self-monitoring, cognitive restructuring, and exposure) to relaxation training and found equivalent effects, though the unified treatment had lower drop-out rates. Unified treatments for co-occurring substance abuse and affective disorders are emerging (Osilla, Hepner, Muñoz, Woo, & Watkins, 2009). This book expands the field of unified, transdiagnostic treatments beyond mental health to substance abuse and health behaviors. It does so by providing an approach to integrating MI, as the foundation for relational factors, with CBT's shared elements. These can be used across different areas of behavior change and symptom remission to improve mental and physical health.

The Spirit of MI

MI is not just a compendium of techniques; it is a style of interacting with people. As such, the foundation of MI is its spirit. According to Miller and Rollnick (2012), the MI spirit consists of four interrelated elements: (1) partnership, (2) acceptance, (3) compassion, and (4) evocation (PACE). *Partnership* is a collaborative, guiding relationship with you and the client side by side instead of one in front of the other. *Acceptance* involves autonomy support by which you emphasize respect for the person's self-determination and freedom of choice. Acceptance also includes expressing accurate empathy and supporting self-efficacy with an inherent appreciation for the person's worth and an affirming stance. *Compassion* is a dedication to promoting the welfare of others, but is distinct from personal feelings of sympathy or personalization of the experience. *Evocation* is the idea that the client has

> MI is not just a compendium of techniques, it is a style of interacting with people.

inherent wisdom and strength for change that you draw out instead of a missing ingredient that you must provide as in CBT approaches.

MI as Four Processes

In addition to the above four elements, MI is organized in terms of four processes: (1) engaging, (2) focusing, (3) evoking, and (4) planning. These elements are meant to be overlapping and not necessarily sequential. All four processes may be present in each session; later we will discuss how all four processes are present in different components of CBT when you work within an integrated MI–CBT approach. The processes are helpful for organizing your thinking about a session.

Engaging is the process of developing rapport with the client and understanding of the client's dilemma. Why is or isn't the person considering change and what is getting in the way? Engaging is the process of establishing the working relationship, the therapeutic alliance. While a strong working alliance is the foundation of any intervention approach and is consistently discussed in the CBT literature, the practitioner communication behaviors necessary to promote alliance and address ruptures in alliance are rarely specified. MI specifies these behaviors.

Focusing is the process by which a practitioner and a client become clear on the direction and goal of the conversation. Often the direction and associated goals are about changing behaviors, but not necessarily so. The focus may be about a choice (e.g., forgiveness, a job change) or about an internal process (e.g., tolerance, acceptance). The process of focusing is more than agenda setting or treatment planning, with a list of goals or tasks. It is the collaborative process of determining the scope of the conversation, which can include goals and tasks as well as thoughts, feelings, and concerns.

Evoking is the process of drawing out the client's own words about change so that the client him- or herself argues for change instead of the practitioner doing it for the client. In the evoking process, you build intrinsic motivation to change the target behavior/concern of focus. In MI, this is done by eliciting and verbally reinforcing change talk with the kind of reflections and affirmations described below. Change is driven by a person's own desire, ability, reasons, or need to change as opposed to those of somebody else. This is central to MI and particularly relevant for CBT. Typically, the provider often presents the rationale for treatment components, presents reasons for why particular skills or relevant homework is important, and/or tries to underscore the negative consequences of current thoughts and behaviors. Yet, most people are more likely to believe what they say themselves compared to what someone else tells them.

Evocation may run counter to the natural instinct to "help" clients by correcting what you construe as flawed reasoning or poor decision making or by imparting unsolicited advice. Miller and Rollnick (2002, 2012) describe this phenomenon as the *righting reflex*, the human tendency to correct things that are perceived as wrong. This tendency often translates into premature problem solving and advice giving, which prevents clients from being actively involved in their own treatment process and leads to other forms of disengagement (e.g., emergence of language against change, avoidance of homework assignments). This is a dilemma for CBT practitioners because education about a mental health problem followed by skills training are typically the key elements of treatment. Motivation for change is a function of how important change is to the client and his or her confidence about making the change. MI skills address both of these components of motivation, and MI skills support the client's own motivation for change even when the provider is sharing relevant information or skills training.

If ambivalence is the balancing between change and the status quo, the *planning* process occurs when the balance begins to tip toward change. The conversation naturally turns to statements about a possible commitment to change and options for a plan of action. Miller and Rollnick (2012) subsume the process of implementing change plans and enacting and maintaining change (the targets of CBT elements) within the planning process.

A Brief Overview of Core MI Skills

MI uses a set of core communication skills, in the spirit of MI, to promote the four processes described above. These skills are asking open questions, affirming, making reflective statements, summarizing, and informing and advising. Reflective statements and open questions are the core skills necessary for MI–CBT integration. We will show you how to use them in different ways for different purposes. Reflective statements are used to communicate accurate empathy and to test your hypotheses about how the client experiences the world. Offering reflections involves stating to the person what you heard, possibly adding an emphasis or meaning. Reflections are also used to reinforce or emphasize components of the conversation for strategic purposes (e.g., to explore ambivalence, to strengthen motivation). Reflective statements can also be affirming because they are reflections of what the person said that emphasize his or her strengths or efforts. You can also use a string of reflections to summarize what the client has said. The string can tie together earlier points, can emphasize the transition from ambivalence to change, and can be used to transition to different components of the session.

While a significant amount of communication can occur from reflective statements alone, open questions can continue to evoke the person's views, concerns, and motivations. In MI, you facilitate conversation with open-ended questions and deemphasize closed-ended questions that elicit a single-word response. Questions and reflections can also be used to provide information and advice in an MI style. In later chapters, you will see how the sequence "ask–tell–ask–reflect" serves this purpose. First, you ask for permission to provide information and elicit the person's interest and knowledge about the topic. Second, you provide information or advice in small, digestible bits. Third, you elicit the client's reaction and reflect the response. This gives you a snapshot of how MI specifies what you say, how you say it, and when you say it. The remaining chapters will show you how to use these communication skills to make CBT work better.

How This Book Is Structured

This guide focuses on the shared elements of the most widely researched CBT approaches such as initiating treatment, assessment and treatment planning, self-monitoring, cognitive and behavioral skills training, promoting homework completion, and maintaining change. A chapter is dedicated to each treatment element, and we present each element in terms of the four MI processes. We do not expect this book to replace MI texts, and consequently MI skills are not presented in as full detail as they would be in an MI-only text. Rather, we refer to MI skills in terms of their integration with CBT; you can refer to MI texts to supplement this information. We utilize examples across multiple behaviors and diagnoses including internalizing symptoms, substance use, and health behaviors. The chapters include activities for your own professional development or for training others (see Activity 1.1 at the end of this chapter). A final chapter reviews future directions including training issues. To demonstrate the unified approach of MI–CBT integration, we intersperse throughout case examples with a range of different target behaviors or problems such as depression, obesity, anxiety, substance abuse, and medication adherence.

MI was never intended to be a comprehensive psychotherapy (Miller & Rollnick, 2009), but rather an approach to behavior change. Yet studies suggest that MI seems to provide a strong foundation for addressing the therapeutic alliance and motivation in the context of other treatments such as CBT. Thus, we support the assertion that MI is not merely a tool for facilitating behavior change but rather has implications for informing psychotherapy in general in the following ways (Miller, 2012). MI emphasizes the belief in the capacity for human growth and change. MI puts the person's choice and decision at the forefront of the therapy encounter. MI promotes acceptance and compassion for ambivalence. Finally, MI supports careful attention to the language of the practitioner and the client, specifying the general relational factors of psychotherapy. As such, MI may be a trellis that supports psychotherapy intervention delivery (Haddock et al., 2012). By integrating MI with the most commonly shared elements of CBT, we use a transdiagnostic approach and advance the implementation of evidence-based practice. Our hope is to reduce the burden on practitioners. Rather than sifting through multiple manuals and sitting through multiple trainings, you may take core factors and elements as specified by MI–CBT integration and promote their application across conditions and settings.

ACTIVITY 1.1 FOR PRACTITIONERS

MI–CBT Integration Card Sort

Integration can take a number of different forms. Treatment integration involves looking beyond the boundaries of single-school approaches to see what can be learned from the theories and techniques of other perspectives (Strickler, 2011). *Technical integration* is when you integrate techniques from different approaches, while *theoretical integration* refers to the process of bringing together concepts from different approaches that may differ in fundamental ways. *Assimilative integration* is a more recent concept that allows you to maintain a solid grounding in one theoretical worldview while incorporating strategies from other approaches. We believe this book could be applicable to your choice of integration.

ACTIVITY GOAL: This activity asks you to consider the theoretical and technical components of MI and CBT and decide the approach to integration that will work best for you as you utilize this guide.

ACTIVITY INSTRUCTIONS: In the table below, place an X over the words you consider to be descriptors of MI, an O over those you consider to be descriptors of CBT, and an X and an O over those for MI–CBT. When you've finished, answer the questions that follow. This activity may also be done as a card sort: copy and cut out each box in the table. Sort MI-only descriptors into one pile, CBT-only descriptors into another pile, and MI–CBT descriptors into a third pile.

Collaborative	Providing feedback	Agenda setting	Problem solving	Therapeutic alliance
Evoking motivation	Asking permission	Exposure	Case formulation	Providing rationales
Triggers	Empathy	Goal oriented	Assessment	Autonomy
Psycho-education	Identifying triggers	Functional analysis	Identifying distorted cognitions	Eliciting feedback

Reflective listening	Making plans for change	Skills training	Identifying antecedents and consequences	Personal growth and responsibility
Homework	Addressing discord	Treatment planning	Reinforcing change language	Eliciting the client's perspective
Menu of options	Guiding	Self-monitoring	Assessment	Outcome oriented
Increasing activities and mastery	Nonjudgmental	Hypothesis testing	Noticing positive emotions	Socratic questioning

Consider the following questions:

1. Where are the natural overlaps between MI and CBT (boxes with X's *and* O's) __

   _____

   _____

   _____

2. Where MI and CBT don't overlap, are these theoretical concepts or techniques and strategies? _____

   _____

   _____

   _____

3. Where can you creatively integrate the theoretical concepts? _____

   _____

   _____

   _____

4. If the concepts do not seem like they can be integrated, how might this affect your use of the strategies? This issue will be important later when you might need to make choices between MI and CBT strategies because integration does not seem feasible. _____

   _____

   _____

   _____

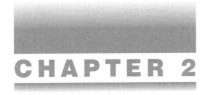

CHAPTER 2

Building Alliance and Motivation at the Onset of Treatment

Ask any practitioner in any field of human services about the critical ingredients of success and you will hear something about the relationship between practitioner and client (e.g., alliance, engagement, collaboration, partnership, patient-centered). Accordingly, in studies, the therapeutic alliance reliably emerges as a strong predictor of behavior change and is consistently cited as a general factor related to successful psychotherapy (Horvath, Del Re, Flückiger, & Symonds, 2011). Studies in medical settings have also demonstrated that practitioners who are informative, provide support and respect for the patient, and facilitate collaboration generally have patients who are more satisfied, are more committed to treatment regimens, and have better health outcomes (Henman, Butow, Brown, Boyle, & Tattersall, 2002; Jahng, Martin, Golin, & DiMatteo, 2005; Kaplan, Greenfield, & Ware Jr., 1989; Ong, De Haes, Hoos, & Lammes, 1995; Stewart et al., 2000; Street Jr., Gordon, & Haidet, 2007; Trummer, Mueller, Nowak, Stidl, & Pelikan, 2006). In a large study of depression treatments (Krupnick et al., 1996), measures of alliance predicted positive treatment outcomes not only for CBT and interpersonal therapy, but also for antidepressant medication and even for placebo medication treatment.

There are two commonly cited definitions of "therapeutic alliance," one focusing on practitioner and client skills and the other focusing on the client's experience. "Alliance" is the ability of the practitioner and the client to work together purposefully to achieve agreed-upon goals (Greenson, 1971). Alliance is also about the client's experience of treatment or of the relationship and whether the practitioner is helpful in achieving the patient's goals (Luborsky, Crits-Christoph,

Alexander, Margolis, & Cohen, 1983). Rogers (1951) placed the onus on the practitioner to achieve a strong alliance, with the alliance itself being the active ingredient of successful psychological treatment. CBT experts note that you must spend enough time developing an alliance at the onset of treatment so that clients will work effectively with you and so that you can maintain the relationship during the challenging work of CBT (Beck, 2011). Thus, this chapter addresses strategies to promote relationship conditions that enable the client to change. You will use these strategies at the onset of treatment to establish a strong alliance and promote treatment retention. Later, we will return to some of these strategies when the alliance ruptures, behavior change falters, or retention drops off during the course of CBT.

In some CBT approaches, the initial sessions focus on assessment and case formulation (Beck, 2011, p. 48), but in MI–CBT these components occur after the initial session tasks described below. We believe, and the evidence suggests (Flynn, 2011; Weiss, Mills, Westra, & Carter, 2013; Westra et al., 2009), that the MI–CBT approach promotes treatment engagement, in addition to increasing motivation for behavior change and session attendance. Clients often feel improved mood and a sense of hope and optimism after experiencing the spirit of MI in the first session. Postpone formal assessment and case formulation until the second session or even longer if the person is not ready to begin CBT. Clients not ready for CBT may be more likely when treatment targets are behaviors that are near and dear to the client (e.g., drinking, eating) compared to client's experiencing significant distress (e.g., depression, anxiety). However, an initial session to solidify the alliance and build motivation for treatment seems to be beneficial in either context (Westra, Constantino, Arkowitz, & Dozois, 2011).

In the rest of this chapter we discuss the uses of the four MI processes—engaging, focusing, evoking, and planning—at the onset of treatment. Recall that these processes do not have to be sequential nor do all four have to be done in a single session. You may also return to different components of this chapter during the course of treatment when you feel motivation has significantly waned. We use the core skills of reflections and open questions to integrate MI and CBT within these four processes.

Engaging

In the process of engagement, you lay the basic groundwork for the session and the course of treatment. Depending on the client, the practitioner–client mix, or the presenting problem, this can occur almost immediately or can take much longer to establish. Engagement may occur more quickly when a client comes for help because of distress and already has significant motivation for change. Often, however, this can take longer to establish when readiness to change behavior is questionable. For example, Carl, a 36-year-old Caucasian male, has been court-ordered for alcohol treatment following a motor vehicle accident and does not really want to be in treatment.

There are at least three tasks for the engagement process in the initial CBT session. First, you probably have information you are required to provide at the onset of treatment (e.g., confidentiality, agency policies) and there are ways to provide this information while simultaneously promoting alliance. Second, you need to understand the client's concerns and why, or why not, the person is considering treatment. Third, you want to explore the client's values and goals as a way to establish rapport and to provide a foundation for later processes. The following sections looks at how to accomplish these tasks using MI.

Opening Exchange

MI is about making every word count. The first statement you offer to the client should immediately promote engagement and demonstrate the MI spirit of collaboration, evocation, compassion, and acceptance. In the opening statement you convey the message that you will support the client's desired changes, rather than direct which changes should be made and how. In "pure" MI you might say, "I am not here to tell you what to change or how to change, but rather to find out what is going on in your life and help you make the changes that you decide to make." However, in MI–CBT you will likely be giving clients information and helping them learn skills about how to change (in an MI style). Thus, it is important to be honest about how treatment will proceed. You might open with something like "I am not here to tell you that you have to change or have to do certain things to change. Instead we can explore your goals and values and together decide what things might be needed to reach your goals."

Now, it is important to find out the client's response. This can be done with a simple pause, but might require an open question to elicit feedback: "What do you think about that approach?" If an open question is too abstract,

> Convey how you will support the client's desired changes, rather than direct which changes should be made and how.

try a multiple-choice question: "Is that what you expected or different from what you expected? Why?" Reflect after every answer to show you are listening and not just interrogating. Recall that reflective statements are used to communicate accurate empathy and to test your hypotheses about how the client experiences the world. Reflections are also used to emphasize or reinforce components of the conversation for strategic purposes (e.g., to highlight strengths, to strengthen motivation). For example, you may be exploring distrust if a client responds with a statement like "Yeah, I heard *that* before," or a client might express concern about whether treatment will be helpful with a response like "I don't even know what I want, so how can you help me?" Alternatively, you may have an opportunity to reinforce hope and optimism if the client responds with something like "Well, that would be different—a nice change." Whatever the client's response, reflections will ensure that you do not miss opportunities to reinforce statements in favor of change, and at a minimum show the client that you are closely paying attention!

> ### TIP for Opening Statement: Avoid Labels
>
> Avoiding labels, diagnoses, or even reducing the use of the term "problem" is important in MI, as all these labels can carry a negative connotation, create feelings of hostility or defensiveness, and decrease self-efficacy to change behaviors. For example, if Carl is labeled as an "alcoholic," he may believe there is little the practitioner can do to alter his drinking, as it is a label that cannot be changed. Overuse of the term "problem" can elicit defensiveness if the client is still ambivalent about whether the target behavior or symptom is a problem at all. Instead, simply name the behavior or symptom: "You were referred to discuss drinking." This helps convey a nonjudgmental attitude, which will promote openness and honesty.

Providing Information: Ask–Tell–Ask

After the opening statement, you often must convey certain information (e.g., the rules of confidentiality, probable length of treatment). Miller and Rollnick (2012) suggest that you sandwich that information between questions and reflections so that you maintain the MI spirit. We call the sandwich ask–tell–ask, or ATA. This strategy is utilized throughout MI–CBT integration, so we briefly address ATA here as an opening strategy. First, *ask* for permission to give information/advice (increases collaboration and supports autonomy) *or* ask clients what they know or want to know (increases evocation, saves you from providing unnecessary information, supports autonomy). The second step is to *tell*—give the client information in small bits. Last, you *ask* the client about his or her point of view regarding the information provided, such as "What is your reaction to that?" or "How does this sound to you?" Reflect the response. As a point of reference, you should not provide more than two or three sentences of information without eliciting the person's thoughts or feelings about that information.

> PRACTITIONER: Celia, if it's OK with you, I would like to tell you about confidentiality. [Ask]
>
> CELIA: Sure.
>
> PRACTITIONER: Well, basically I won't share information you tell me unless it's about hurting yourself or someone else. And in those situations, we would talk about who I would need to tell and exactly what I would tell them. [Tell] What do you think of that? [Ask]

CELIA: Well, I guess that makes sense. What do you mean by hurting myself?

PRACTITIONER: You're wondering when I might have to tell someone. [Reflect] If you told me that you were going to do something that put your life in danger, we would have to make a plan to tell someone else in your life to keep you safe. [Tell] What's your reaction to that? [Ask]

Another type of information usually provided at the beginning of a session is how the session will proceed. This typically sounds something like, "Today I'd like to find out more about what brought you here and tell you a little bit about my approach." In CBT, sessions often begin with a formal session agenda (Beck, 2011, p. 60). In MI, the term "agenda setting" refers to a process of focusing on treatment targets (see below). For MI–CBT integration, we suggest beginning every session by collaboratively setting the agenda for the remainder of the session using ATA. Begin to model this process in the very first session even when formal CBT tasks are not yet occurring. As demonstrated in the following example, you want to (1) ask for permission, (2) state planned session components, (3) elicit feedback, (4) reflect the client's feedback, and (5) ask the client what he or she would like to add.

PRACTITIONER: If it's OK with you, [Ask permission] I'd like to discuss what we will cover today. I'd like to find out more about what brought you here today, decide what your goals are, and talk about the kinds of things we can do in future sessions to help with your goals if you decide to continue. [Tell] How does that sound to you? [Ask]

CARL: I guess that's fine, but I really didn't want to come here.

PRACTITIONER: This was something you felt forced to do. [Reflect] I definitely want to hear more about that. What would you like to add to what we cover today? [Open question for collaborative agenda setting]

CARL: Nothing really, but I want to make sure you sign the papers I need for probation.

PRACTITIONER: OK, you need to make sure you're meeting your probation requirements. [Reflect] I'll add that to the agenda and make sure we don't forget at the end.

Understanding the Client's Dilemma, Values, and Goals

After the opening exchange and the initial tasks of treatment, now is the time to truly listen. In MI, you actively listen with the MI skills of reflections and open questions to promote accurate empathy and to test hypotheses about the client's world. Gordon (1970) described 12 roadblocks to active listening that interfere with client self-exploration and practitioner understanding in the engagement phase:

1. Ordering, directing, or commanding
2. Warning, cautioning, or threatening
3. Telling people what they should do; moralizing
4. Disagreeing, judging, criticizing, or blaming
5. Generic approving or praising
6. Shaming, ridiculing, or labeling
7. Interpreting or analyzing
8. Reassuring, sympathizing, or consoling
9. Withdrawing, distracting, humoring, or changing the subject
10. Persuading with logic, arguing, or lecturing
11. Giving advice, making suggestions, or providing solutions
12. Questioning or probing.

Note that in MI–CBT integration there is a time and place for roadblocks 11 and 12, but these practitioner behaviors can interfere with the engagement process, particularly in the first session, and even more so if you have not firmly agreed on specific goals for treatment. The last roadblock, questioning or probing, requires clarification. While listening involves primarily reflections, an open question may be necessary to continue the conversation. Closed questions (which yield yes or no answers) do not continue the conversation and can sound more like probing, particularly when asked in a series. To avoid probing, questions should be sandwiched with reflections. See how in the exchange below there are at least twice as many reflections as questions, which is an overall goal of MI communication.

PRACTITIONER: Carl, tell me about how you got here today. [Open question]

CARL: Well, my probation officer said I had to show up.

PRACTITIONER: So you were forced to come. [Reflect]

CARL: Yeah, well my choices are kind of limited right now.

PRACTITIONER: You feel like you have no choice. [Reflect]

CARL: Yeah, well if I don't come here, I won't get off probation.

PRACTITIONER: Getting off probation is your main goal right now. [Reflect]

CARL: Yeah. [Reflect]

PRACTITIONER: What needs to happen for you to reach that goal? [Open question]

CARL: Well, apparently I need to quit drinking, but I really don't see that happening. [Dilemma]

PRACTITIONER: You need to quit drinking to reach your goal of getting off probation, but that kind of change is hard to imagine. [Reflect]

CARL: Exactly!

Other questions that can move the conversation forward include:

"Walk me through a typical day."
"Who are the most important people in your life right now?"
"How do you hope your life will be different a year from now?"
"If you were to pick a motto for how you live your life, what would it be?"
"What would you say your top three values are?" (You can offer a written list of values on a sheet or on cards).

Reflect each answer!

> **TIP for Listening: Avoid Turning Reflections into Questions**
>
> The inflection, your tone of voice (i.e., turning it up into a question or stating it in a neutral tone in a flat-sounding statement) at the end of a statement, can make or break the impact of your reflection. Your goal should be to maintain a neutral, steady inflection in your use of reflections because they can easily be turned into closed questions with a rising inflection at the end. For example, if a client describes his drinking frequency and you respond, "You drank a case of beer [high inflection]?," the client may feel judged because you sound surprised and even disappointed. Try this out loud and see how it sounds. However, if you lower the inflection to sound straightforward and matter-of-fact—"You drank a case of beer"—you express understanding of the client's dilemma.

Sustain Talk and Discord

Trouble in the alliance and in the course of treatment in general has historically been referred to as "resistance." In the early days of psychotherapy, resistance was conceptualized as a negative patient state or even trait. More recently, resistance in psychotherapy has been reconceptualized as an interpersonal process affected by both client and practitioner variables (Engle & Arkowitz, 2006; Freeman & McCluskey, 2005).

Miller and Rollnick (2012) further clarify these concepts. They note that when practitioners feel they are struggling with an individual not ready for change, they often describe this process as resistance. However, language against changing and statements in favor of sustaining the target behavior are a normal part of ambivalence. Thus, MI distinguishes between "sustain talk" and "discord." Discord is about the relationship. It is akin to disharmony in the collaboration or ruptures in alliance.

Reflections can go a long way in responding to both sustain talk and discord. Other strategies to reduce sustain talk include a review of the cons of behavior change with empathy and nonjudgment followed by a review of the pros. Humans have a tendency to experience negative feelings (i.e., psychological reactance) when they perceive their personal freedoms are limited or controlled (Brehm, 1966). Emphasizing autonomy can reduce sustain talk. You directly acknowledge or emphasize the client's freedom of choice and personal responsibility. "You're right. Nobody can force you to change"; "You're the one who knows yourself best here. What do you think ought to be on this change plan?" This last statement moves from addressing sustain talk to eliciting language in favor of change, "change talk" (see "Evoking" below).

When you experience discord, your overall goal is to do something different! Miller and Rollnick (2012) identify three specific strategies to respond to discord: apologizing, affirming, and shifting focus. Apologizing is a simple "I'm sorry," specifying your potential role in the discord: "I'm sorry if I was lecturing"; "I'm sorry if I didn't understand." If you are not sure exactly what you did, you can apologize about your recognition that the client feels discord: "I'm sorry you're feeling frustrated." As noted in Chapter 1, affirming statements are reflections of positive qualities or strengths in the person: "You keep persisting with trying therapy even though you're not sure anyone can help you." Finally, shifting focus is simply steering the conversation to a less controversial topic. Options for shifting focus may include a discussion of other areas of the person's life that may be related to behavior change or to an intermediary goal.

Focusing

In the engagement process, you and your client agree to go on a trip, in the focusing process you clarify *where* you are going. You may not draw the details of the map (that occurs later during case conceptualization and treatment planning), but you and your client collaboratively determine the destination and agree (at least tentatively) that CBT is the way to get you there. Bordin (1979) notes that therapeutic alliance is not just the positive bond that develops between client and practitioner but also is agreement about the tasks of treatment.

> In the engagement process, you and your client agree to go on a trip; in the focusing process you clarify where you are going.

In the process of focusing, the practitioner becomes the guide for the client on this journey. Miller and Rollnick (2012) describe a guiding communication style as one that sits in the middle of the continuum between following and directing. In a *following style,* you mostly listen and keep questions, informing, or advising to a minimum. In a *directing style,* you are mostly informing, asking some questions, and doing a minimum of listening. In a *guiding style,* you listen, ask, and inform in relatively equal balance. You can see how this style is consistent with the three core skills of reflecting, asking open questions, and providing information with ask–tell–ask.

When focusing, there are three possible scenarios. First, there may be no general focus. In that case, you can return to the engaging process, with a particular emphasis on exploring values and goals to provide a general focus, and then move on to a structured conversation to develop more specific treatment targets. For example, Sam is a 19-year-old, Caucasian, heterosexual young male college student who has social anxiety disorder and struggles about making friends at school and meeting young women to date. He is quite isolated in that he does not really have friends and can get depressed, particularly on weekends when he sees other students making their plans with one another. On the rare occasion that he tries to go to a party on the school campus, he tends to drink alcohol heavily as a way to reduce his anxiety in hopes it will help him talk to people, but typically this results in too much drinking and intoxication to be an effective strategy. He rarely, if ever, participates in class at school, and avoids taking any class that would require him to give a presentation. There was an initial agreement that Sam needed treatment for the distress he was feeling; he knew that he did not like the way his life was going. However, the specific focus of treatment was unclear: social anxiety, depression, or alcohol use? After some discussion, the collaboratively developed focus was on the social anxiety, which he (and the therapist in terms of the case conceptualization) believed drove the symptoms of depression and excessive alcohol use.

Alternatively, the focus may be clear based on the setting, such as with Carl who is court-ordered for alcohol treatment. Sometimes the focus is clear based on your expertise, but the client may not yet have considered this focus. For example, Celia is a 40-year-old Caucasian woman. She lives with her husband and adolescent daughter. Her marriage is crumbling in large part because of her symptoms of irritability and inactivity. She has some comorbid anxiety and reports spending a lot of her time worrying about something happening to her family or her own safety, particularly around driving. Celia comes to see you because her marriage is failing but in the engagement process it is clear she is struggling with depression. Now that you have developed rapport, you may provide that suggestion with ATA. "I know you came here wanting help with your relationship, but some other ideas come to mind based on our discussions so far. Would it be OK to discuss these?" Once you have the client's permission, you may suggest, "We have been talking about your struggles with depression, and I am wondering if we might talk about how depression interferes with your relationships. What do you think?" In the spirit of MI, the client can veto the suggestion or ask to address both concerns, and then you can negotiate a shared agenda with reflections and open questions.

In the last scenario, there are multiple possible treatment goals, and you and your client must zoom in on a starting point. It could be there are multiple concerns, and the client is overwhelmed about where to start (e.g., depression, anxiety, marijuana use, marital conflict). It could also be that there are multiple steps that are necessary for the client to achieve the desired outcome. A good place to start is a summarizing reflection where you string together reflections of the engagement conversation and ask for permission to develop a shared agenda. For example, "We have talked about several things that are important to you such as being less depressed and anxious, getting along better with your husband, your job situation, and how sleeping pills might play a role in all this. Would it be OK with you if we now discuss where to focus our sessions together?" Now you have several options. If the client's story suggests that one behavior is clearly driving the rest, then feel free to offer information or advice with ATA. Alternatively, you may ask the client which behavior he or she would like to start with. Another option is to begin with the behavior that seems least difficult to overcome so that the client can increase self-efficacy, and then target more difficult behaviors.

What about targeting multiple behaviors simultaneously? There is limited research on multiple behavior change, but the most recent review (Prochaska & Prochaska, 2011) suggested that outcomes for studies targeting diet and physical activity simultaneously were disappointing, but targeting two addictions simultaneously (including smoking) yielded more long-term sobriety from alcohol and illicit drugs. In the area of disease prevention, multiple behavior change interventions were more successful for cancer prevention than for cardiovascular risk. There are no data indicating how many behaviors should be targeted simultaneously, though most studies did not tackle more than two. Only four studies were identified that compared sequential versus simultaneous behavior change and the results were inconclusive. Thus, without strong evidence to date, we believe that relying on collaborative decision making is the best option.

TIP for Focusing: Use a Visual Tool

A Focusing Map (Miller & Rollnick, 2012, pp. 109–110; Rollnick, Miller, & Butler, 2008) is a visual collaborative tool where together you draw circles representing different parts of the client's values, goals, and dilemmas. The circles can be different sizes to represent their level of importance. You can utilize arrows to represent which concerns trigger other concerns and allow a focus on the more proximal rather than distal concerns (see Client Handout 2.1*; the map can also be drawn from scratch with a client so that various circles can overlap as needed). Figure 2.1 shows a Focusing Map for Celia.

---

*All reproducible client handouts are at the ends of chapters.

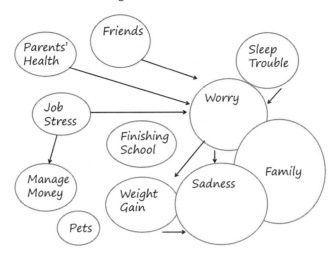

FIGURE 2.1. Focusing Map for Celia.

Evoking

Once there is a change goal in mind, the heart of MI is evoking the client's intrinsic motivation for change. You do this by using open questions and reflections to elicit and reinforce "change talk." These are client statements in favor of change or against sustaining current behavior. These statements indicate desire, ability, reasons, or need to change. The strongest change talk uses commitment language such as "I am ready . . ." and "I am going to. . . ." When initiating treatment, you want to elicit and reinforce change talk about the target behavior(s) determined in the focusing process, but it is also critical to elicit and reinforce change talk about attending in CBT. Try Activity 2.1 at the end of the chapter for practice.

> The heart of MI is evoking the client's intrinsic motivation for change.

Eliciting and Reinforcing Change Talk about Target Behaviors

Throughout the engaging and focusing processes, you should be listening for change talk. In MI, change talk is "reinforced" by responding with reflections and asking for elaboration.

Mary is a 14-year-old African American female with primary obesity (not secondary to another medical condition). She lives with her mother and two younger brothers. Her mother has enrolled Mary in a weight loss program. In the following dialogue, see how the practitioner reinforces Mary's change talk about weight loss even in the context of ambivalence:

MARY: My mother hassles me all the time, and it's not as easy as she thinks. If she got off my back I might do a lot better, [Ability to change] but the arguments we have are just too much, they just make me want to eat more.

PRACTITIONER: You might do a lot better with following an eating plan if you and your mother would stop fighting. [Reflect ability]

MARY: Yeah, all day long she nags me about what I'm eating. It makes me want to just quit this whole thing, but I really want to lose some weight before summer. [Desire for change]

PRACTITIONER: Tell me more about why you want to lose weight before summer. [Open question to elaborate change talk]

MARY: All the kids hang out outside in shorts and t-shirts. When it is hot, I don't like to go outside because I don't want to wear clothes to show my fat. [Reasons for change]

PRACTITIONER: You want to lose weight so that you can go outside and be with the other kids. [Reflect reasons for change] What would it be like to be more comfortable in your own skin? [Open question for elaboration]

MARY: Well, it's hard to imagine because I never have been. And usually I don't care. I have enough friends. But I need to lose weight if I'm ever going to be comfortable at least in the summer. [Need for change]

Sometimes reflections and asking for elaboration are enough to elicit more change talk and evoking occurs naturally throughout the engaging and focusing process. Other times, it feels like pulling teeth. If the conversation does not automatically tilt toward change talk, the open questions below will help you to evoke more of this language of motivation. Of course, as before, you will reflect the client's responses and ask for further elaboration when appropriate.

Perhaps the most direct way to elicit change talk is to ask for it—for example: "If you decided to make a change, how would you do it?"; "Why would you want to reduce the virus in your blood?"; "How would things be better for you if you had more energy?" You can also tailor questions to elicit change talk based on what you already have learned about the client. For example, you might say to Mary, "You mentioned earlier that you tend to eat more when your mother fights with you. What do you think needs to change here?"

Inquiring about how important people in the client's life perceive the target concern can elicit change talk in clients who do not necessarily see a need for change. However, you want to emphasize your interest in your clients' ideas and not what others have told them: "Everyone is telling you what needs to change. What do *you* want? What part of your life feels less than perfect for you right now?"

Other types of questions can elicit change talk when direct questions are not enough or when a client is highly ambivalent and direct questions seem too insistent. Imagining questions include asking the client to look into the future and imagine life if the client made a change or to look back to a time when the target behaviors were not interfering with the client's life. Imagining extremes is an adaptation of this approach: "What's the worst thing that might happen if you continue drinking?" and "What's the best thing that might happen if you decided to take your medication every day?"

Values questions explore incongruities between your client's values and goals with the current behavior. By actively listening, you may already have clues to values that you can use,

For example, Eugene is a 23-year-old Latino male who was diagnosed with HIV 1 year ago. He believes he contracted it from his previous boyfriend who was 10 years his senior and is now incarcerated. He is currently living with an aunt because his parents asked him to leave the home after high school when they found out he was gay. He recently disclosed his HIV status to his aunt. He currently works at a fast food restaurant and takes one culinary class at a local community college. He started antiretroviral treatment about 9 months ago, but stopped in the last month as he missed his last medical visit and ran out of medications.

Eugene's practitioner uses a values question. "It is really important to you to be independent. I wonder how taking care of your health might help you be more independent." Eugene might reply, "If I get sick, I'll have to rely on other people more."

For Carl you might say, "This probation has really interfered with your independence. How would changing your drinking get your independence back?" For Celia this might sound like, "Your marriage is clearly your priority. How would improving your mood improve your marriage?" You can also discuss how change has to be done in such a way that it does not interfere with a client's values. For example, Mary values include having fun with her friends, but a weight loss program could interfere with that value if she has to eat differently from everyone else. Asking Mary how a weight loss plan could accommodate those values can elicit change talk. "I wonder if there is a meal plan that would allow you to go out with friends and go to restaurants." Mary might respond, "If I could just work on smaller portions of the foods I like, or finding healthy foods on the menu, I bet I could follow it a lot better."

Finally, questions about personal strengths can support self-efficacy and elicit change talk about ability. You can encourage stories regarding past change successes either directly related to the target behavior or to other difficult changes. Similarly, you can inquire about successfully accomplished goals from the past, personal strengths, or social supports available to help with overcoming challenges (e.g., "Who helped you?"; "What are the things you did that made a difference?").

Eliciting and Reinforcing Change Talk for Session Attendance

While eliciting and reinforcing change talk about the target behavior may be sufficient for an MI-only approach, in MI–CBT integration you will need to elicit and reinforce change talk for ongoing session attendance (and later for treatment tasks). The strategies above can all be used to focus on session attendance instead of the target behavior (e.g., "Why did you feel you needed to come here today?"; "How does attending sessions help you reach your goal and be more independent?"; "How would attending sessions help you meet your goal of improving your marriage?"). An additional strategy that is also a central component of CBT is providing the treatment rationale, addressing the CBT model of the etiology of the target concerns, and explaining the approach to intervention. Client's acceptance of the treatment rationale has consistently predicted treatment outcome (Addis & Carpenter, 2000).

In CBT, providing the rationale might sound something like this:

> "We are going to be using an approach called cognitive-behavioral therapy—or CBT—to help with your problems. The basic idea in CBT is that how we think affects how we feel and also what we do. So we will meet weekly to work on identifying situations that trigger certain thoughts and then discuss how to manage those thoughts to change how we feel and behave. Does that make sense?"

In an MI–CBT approach, you would not *provide* the rationale but rather you would *discuss* the rationale using MI skills while evoking motivation for attending sessions. In the example of Eugene below, the practitioner discusses the rationale with ATA and reflections. You are eliciting reasons for session attendance while emphasizing autonomy with "you" statements. Note that the word "problem" is avoided. Using the term "CBT" is not necessary though it is not contraindicated.

> PRACTITIONER: Based on what we have talked about so far, you decided your goal is to improve your health by taking your medication consistently. [Reflect from focusing and emphasize autonomy with "you"] How do you see meeting with me as helping to achieve that goal? [Ask]
>
> EUGENE: Well, I really don't know because just talking about it doesn't seem to help.
>
> PRACTITIONER: So you've noticed that simply talking about your goals isn't enough. [Reflect] In the kind of work I do, our sessions focus on how situations, thoughts, feelings, and behaviors go together. [Tell] What is an example about how a situation, thought, or feeling affected taking your medications? [Ask]

EUGENE: I don't know what you mean.

PRACTITIONER: Well, some people find that when they are in certain places or when they are feeling or thinking a certain way they are more likely to miss taking medications. [Tell]

EUGENE: Oh, yeah, I usually miss when I sleep over my boyfriend's house, and sometimes I skip because I don't feel like dealing with having HIV.

PRACTITIONER: You can already think of a situation or a thought or feeling when you are more likely to miss your HIV meds. [Affirming reflection] In our sessions we wouldn't just talk about them, but we would work on skills to help you change the way you manage different situations and the thoughts and feelings that affect your behavior. [Tell] What do you think about that approach? [Ask]

EUGENE: I guess it makes sense, but what do you mean by skills?

PRACTITIONER: The idea of working on thoughts, feelings and behaviors, and how you respond to different situations makes sense to you, but you're not sure what working on skills means. [Reflect] What it means is that we would practice strategies to cope with situations or change behaviors in sessions, and then you would try things out on your own between sessions. When we meet the next time, we would discuss how that went and see whether we need more practice or to try something different. [Tell] So now what does working on skills mean to you? [Ask]

EUGENE: I guess it means that you will teach me stuff to change things.

PRACTITIONER: Yes, I could give you suggestions if it makes sense for your life and fits with what you want to change. [Emphasize autonomy]

EUGENE: I guess I could try that. Do I have to come every week forever? Because it's not like I have mental problems.

PRACTITIONER: You can see how skills can help you, but you're not sure how often you have to come or for how long, especially because mental health issues are not your concern. [Reflect] Ideally, if we work together every week, we can make the most progress, especially if the skills are new or you're finding your goal hard to reach. [Tell] Why do you think weekly sessions would be best for making progress? [Ask]

EUGENE: I guess because I am more likely to practice and less likely to forget.

PRACTITIONER: The more often you practice the skills, the more likely you are to make them a habit. [Reflect with some tell] How long we meet really depends on where you are with reaching your goal. [Tell] How does that answer your question? [Ask]

Planning

You may transition to the planning process when you feel you are hearing sufficient change talk indicating that the person is on board with continuing treatment. Alternatively, you may transition toward the end of the session (e.g., when there are only about 10 minutes left) with an ambivalent client, and you want to plan for the client to return for at least one more visit. Using a string of reflections, summarize the discussion so far as a way of transitioning to planning. This summary first synthesizes the ambivalence discussions, highlights the change talk, and ends with a key question. In the case of Celia, you might summarize in this manner:

> Using a string of reflections, summarize the discussion as a way of transitioning to planning.

> "We have talked about a lot of different things in terms of your marriage, your activity level, and your mood. You are ready for a change and do not want things to continue as they are. You're worried about how much work it will take to be less depressed and you want to make sure your marriage doesn't fall apart while you work on that. You're not sure whether your husband will come to sessions, but you are willing to come every week if you can see some changes pretty quickly. So what do you think you'll do next?"

Key questions are focused on guiding the client to explore how he or she might go about change and engage in the next steps.

MI emphasizes the formation of a change plan with sufficient detail to increase the likelihood of success, while continuing to evoke motivation so that engagement is not lost. The first step is setting a goal that includes both the target behavior and session attendance, but if the person is not ready to change at all, a session attendance goal alone is sufficient. In Carl's case, he is not ready to commit to quitting drinking, so his goal is to follow his probation requirements, which include short-term sobriety and weekly session attendance.

Using reflections, questions, and ATA to provide information, advice, or a menu of options for change, you guide the client to delineate steps to reach the goal (e.g., recording the next appointment, managing transportation, developing a strategy to avoid forgetting) and you review reasons to reach the goal based on the discussions so far (remembering to elicit the reasons and reinforce them with reflections!). Finally, it is critical to identify potential barriers and decide on what to do to overcome them (if–then plans)—for example: "*If* my babysitter is ill, *then* I will ask my mother to watch the baby. I will talk to her ahead of time to see if she can be my backup in emergencies." Do not hesitate to use your expertise (with permission) and offer options for these potential barriers. Similarly, if there are barriers that you are concerned about that have not yet been identified, you may use ATA to present them to the client:

"If it's OK with you, I wanted to mention some other barriers that I have seen before. Some clients have told me that they don't want to come to sessions when they don't feel like dealing with their problems. How do you think that might apply to you?"

The change plan can be done as a verbal transaction, but the act of writing down the plan (see Client Handout 2.2) to encode the intention may increase the likelihood of implementation (Gollwitzer, 1999). Alternatively, you can record the plan for the client and leave a copy with him or her at the end of the session. After the change plan steps are completed, you affirm the client's ideas, boost self-efficacy with statements of hope and optimism, and end with a summary of the discussion.

In the case of Sam, his three presenting concerns (not having friends and being anxious in social situations, feeling depressed, and using alcohol to excess) seemed to all relate back to social anxiety. Although he seemed to understand this, a potential barrier to change involved his anxiety about engaging in exposures. Hence, his goals were to decrease anxiety so that he could make friends, which would lead to reduced depression and not as great a need to binge drink when he was in social situations. Sam's completed Change Plan is shown in Figure 2.2. The practitioner develops a final summary that affirms client's ideas, emphasizes change talk, expresses hope, and emphasizes autonomy using "you" statements: "You have some good reasons to consider treatment for social anxiety even though it may be stressful. You see how attending sessions and gradually exposing yourself to fearful situations might help you to achieve your goals, and you were very creative in coming up with ways to overcome possible barriers. I am hopeful that we can work together and achieve the goals you set out for yourself."

TIP for Change Plans: Use Strategies to Elicit Commitment Language

Open-ended questions that directly elicit language about commitment and taking steps can consolidate commitment to treatment (e.g., "Why do you feel attending sessions is something you must do?"; "Why do you feel now is the time to see someone and make a change?"). As described above, always reinforce the answers with reflections and questions to promote elaboration. Another strategy is the use of a commitment scaling question or ruler (see Client Handout 2.3). Here you ask the client to rate how committed he or she is to the plan and then ask why the client chose that answer and not something lower (e.g., "You said 'sort of committed,' why sort of versus not committed at all?") to elicit change talk. Note that if you ask why not a higher rating, you will elicit counterchange talk.

PRACTITIONER: So you have a lot of ideas about how to get to sessions regularly. How sure are you that you are going to follow through with this plan? Sort of sure, very sure, or totally sure?

CARL: I am pretty sure I will do it.

PRACTITIONER: Pretty sure. [Reflection] What makes you pretty sure versus something less? [Open question to elicit commitment as opposed to asking "versus something more," which would elicit counterchange talk]

CARL: Well, I know I will get in more trouble if I don't, and I really want my independence back.

PRACTITIONER: So this plan is something you are pretty sure you will follow through on because *you* think it is important for your future. [Reflect to emphasize autonomy]

My Plan

Changes I would like to make:

Be able to make friends

Not be so anxious initiating conversations with people

Decrease my depressed mood

These changes are important to me because:

I do not want to be on my own forever

I want to have a girlfriend

I do not like how I act when I am drunk

I do not want to be lonely

I plan to take these steps (what, where, when, how):

Try to do behavior therapy for anxiety

Attend sessions and discuss exposures no matter how they go

IF this gets in the way	THEN try this
I am too anxious to try an exposure	Talk to Dr. Steven about working on something lower on the fear hierarchy
I don't want to come to sessions	Try to remember the reasons I want to change, and that I can talk to Dr. Steven about why I didn't want to come
I feel upset and therefore do not want to try any of the home practice	Try to remember the reasons I am doing this treatment (see above)

FIGURE 2.2. Sam's Change Plan.

MI–CBT Dilemmas

What are the dilemmas facing the practitioner integrating MI and CBT in the initial sessions? That is, where are MI and CBT potentially at odds here? In MI you would continue with building motivation and potentially postpone planning and action if the client is not yet "ready." However, ambivalence may not fully resolve before engaging in CBT. We suggest that while you may spend more than a session or two on building motivation before a client is ready to move to the next steps, at some point you need to suggest moving on to the next steps in CBT. If the ambivalence is severe, the client may need to return to treatment at a later date. During subsequent CBT sessions, when ambivalence interferes with progress, you continue to engage, focus, and evoke motivation for changing target behaviors and attending sessions.

Another dilemma is related to organizational requirements. Are there certain things required with regard to paperwork or assessment that must happen during the first session? These requirements could interfere with engagement. While, ideally, any requirements could occur after the first visit, we suggest considering spending at least 10 to 15 minutes on engagement before attending to the necessary agency or protocol requirements. If an intake assessment is necessary before any further treatment contact, consider balancing reflections and questions and review strategies discussed in the next chapter.

================= **ACTIVITY 2.1 FOR PRACTITIONERS** =================

Sequences: Eliciting and Reinforcing Change Talk for Session Attendance

As described above, "change talk" refers to language about desire, ability, reasons, need, and commitment for changing the target behavior and attending sessions. You elicit change talk with targeted open questions. You reinforce change talk with reflections and asking for elaboration if reflections aren't enough to continue the conversation. Thus, when listening to MI-based conversations you should hear sequences like this: (1) practitioner question; (2) client change talk; and (3) practitioner reinforcement with reflection and possibly a follow-up question.

ACTIVITY GOAL: This activity promotes the recognition of these sequences and practice of practitioner strategies to elicit and reinforce change talk.

ACTIVITY INSTRUCTIONS: Following the three samples, fill in the blanks on Items 1–6, making up the details of the case as necessary. You will practice completing each of the three components of the sequences. In the first section, you will complete one of the three components of the sequence (question to elicit change talk, client change talk, reflection of change talk). In the second section, you will use your creativity to complete two of the three components.

Sample A

- **Practitioner Strategy to Elicit Change Talk:** What brought you here today?
- **Client Change Talk:** Well, my mother signed me up for this.
- **Practitioner Reinforcement (Reflection/Question):** *You came to get your mother off your back. How would things be better if that happened?*

Sample B

- **Practitioner Strategy to Elicit Change Talk:** Thinking about the future, how might these sessions improve your marriage?
- **Client Change Talk:** *Well, if you could help me have more energy, I might be able to join my husband in some of his hobbies.*
- **Practitioner Reinforcement (Reflection/Question):** If working on depression gave you more energy,bthat would improve your marriage.

Sample C

- **Practitioner Strategy to Elicit Change Talk:** *Looking back, tell me about a time when you did cut down on drinking.*
- **Client Change Talk:** I quit drinking once before when I was training for a 10K.
- **Practitioner Reinforcement (Reflection/Question):** So a plan that includes an exercise goal is something that might work for you.

Your Turn!

Item 1

- **Practitioner Strategy to Elicit Change Talk:** Why is getting healthier something you need to do?
- **Client Change Talk:** Because I am tired of feeling sick and I don't want to pass anything on to my boyfriend.
- **Practitioner Reinforcement (Reflection/Question):** _____

_____

_____

Item 2

- **Practitioner Strategy to Elicit Change Talk:** What has your wife said about your drinking?
- **Client Change Talk:** _____

_____

_____

- **Practitioner Reinforcement:** Cutting back on drinking may have some effects on your marriage.

Item 3

- **Practitioner Strategy to Elicit Change Talk:** _____
  _____

  _____

- **Client Change Talk:** I think working on how to manage stress could be helpful.
- **Practitioner Reinforcement:** You can see these sessions working for you if we can improve stress management.

Item 4

- **Practitioner Strategy to Elicit Change Talk:** You said that taking care of your family is the most important thing right now. If we worked together on being less depressed, how would that help you reach that goal?
- **Client Change Talk:** _____
  _____

  _____

- **Practitioner Reinforcement:** _____
  _____

  _____

Item 5

- **Practitioner Strategy to Elicit Change Talk:** _____
  _____

  _____

- **Client Change Talk:** _I guess if you helped me in here to get off probation I could get back on my feet._
- **Practitioner Reinforcement:** _____
  _____

  _____

Item 6

- **Practitioner Strategy to Elicit Change Talk:** _____
  _____

  _____

- **Client Change Talk:** _____
  _____

  _____

- **Practitioner Reinforcement:** You really want to wear different types of clothes, and losing some weight will help you reach that goal.

Focusing Map Form

Fill in the circles to represent values, goals, dilemmas, or important relationships and settings, with larger circles representing higher levels of importance.

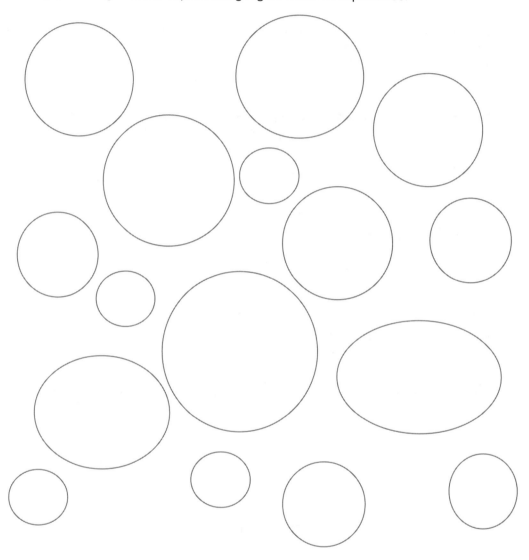

Adapted from Rosengren (2009). Copyright © 2009 The Guilford Press.

Change Plan

My Plan

Changes I would like to make:

_____

_____

_____

_____

These changes are important to me because:

_____

_____

_____

_____

_____

_____

I plan to take these steps (what, where, when, how):

_____

_____

_____

_____

_____

_____

IF this gets in the way	THEN try this
_____	_____
_____	_____
_____	_____
_____	_____
_____	_____

Commitment Ruler

On a scale from 1 to 10, where 1 is "not at all committed" and 10 is "extremely committed," how committed are you to attending weekly sessions to help you make the changes you want to make?

1	2	3	4	5	6	7	8	9	10
Not at all committed				Somewhat committed			Extremely committed		

You chose a _____. List three reasons why you chose this number and not a *lower* number.

1. _____

   _____

   _____

   _____

2. _____

   _____

   _____

   _____

3. _____

   _____

   _____

   _____

CHAPTER 3

Evaluation and Treatment Planning

After the tasks of the initial sessions (developing a therapeutic alliance, understanding the client's dilemma, determining the focus of treatment, building motivation, and planning for treatment participation) are complete, the next step is to flesh out the assessment, case formulation, and treatment plan, though client ambivalence about behavior change may still remain. We discuss the evaluation, case formulation, and development of a treatment plan in a single chapter in the context of the four processes. However, these treatment tasks may or may not occur in a single session because, as noted previously, the processes are not sequential but overlapping. You may prefer to take time between sessions to process the information obtained during evaluation or to discuss the information with a supervisor or team before discussing a treatment plan with the client. If this is the case, you may decide to complete the evaluation and initial case conceptualization in one session while continuing to build motivation for treatment participation, but wait until the next session to address a specific treatment plan while continuing to promote engagement.

The purpose of the initial assessment in CBT is to obtain enough information to collaboratively develop an initial treatment plan, realizing that you and the client will be sharing information and potentially revising the plan on an ongoing basis. In the traditional cognitive model (Beck, 2011, pp. 29–39), situations and events lead to automatic thoughts, which in turn lead to emotional, behavioral, and physiological reactions. In turn, these reactions lead to continued negative automatic thoughts, and a cycle ensues to maintain the presenting problem. These automatic thoughts define how you construe a situation and determine how you will react, and they are influenced by beliefs—both core beliefs and intermediary ones (attitudes, rules, and assumptions). Thus, the purpose of the CBT assessment is to delineate the interplay of these factors. Breaking the cycle involves learning to think and behave more adaptively (and realistically) about the presenting situations, and hence changing the beliefs that drive the automatic thoughts and subsequent reactions. The form of CBT that emphasizes behavioral activation involves helping clients engage in pleasurable activities or activities that promote mastery, to reduce avoidance and break a cycle that causes negative emotions (Martell, Dimidjian, & Herman-Dunn, 2010, p. 197). Hence, the evaluation and treatment planning sessions would involve an analysis of the client's daily and weekly routines and how they are associated with the treatment goals.

Many CBT approaches utilize a functional assessment (Martell et al., 2010, pp. 64–69; Miller, Moyers, Arciniega, Ernst, & Forcehimes, 2005; Naar-King et al., 2016; Parsons, Golub, Rosof, & Holder, 2007). The purpose of a functional assessment is to understand the antecedents and consequences of the target behaviors or the symptoms of concern in terms of the five W's: why, what, where, when, and who. For example, there might be specific places, or people, or times of day that trigger a drinking episode, an eating episode, a depressed mood, or a tendency to miss medications. Alternatively, there may be thoughts, feelings, behaviors, or physiological symptoms that precede or follow engagement in the target behavior or the experience of emotional distress. It is important to analyze the antecedents and consequences in terms of engaging in the target behavior (experiencing distress) and avoiding the target behavior (experiencing stress reduction). By understanding the client's antecedents and consequences, you can explore his or her strengths and resources, the results of which will be used in developing an individual plan for treatment and change.

Engaging

During the initial evaluation phase of treatment, the therapeutic alliance is fragile and can easily be ruptured if the client feels interrogated or if sensitive areas are questioned too quickly. *Proceed with caution.* This is why CBT practitioners often consider the assessment phase to be "pretreatment." In MI, and MI-informed CBT, we believe that every interaction "counts" and is an opportunity to engage the client in treatment and to build motivation for behavior change. Thus the evaluation and treatment planning process is an intervention strategy in its own right.

> During the initial evaluation, the therapeutic alliance is fragile and can easily be ruptured if the client feels interrogated.

Opening Exchange

Three components are a routine part of engagement for the evaluation session as well as subsequent MI–CBT sessions: checking in on the client's previous change plan, setting the session's agenda, and discussing the rationale for the session's objectives.

Checking In

Regardless of the intervention modality, most practitioners typically begin each session by "checking in" on how the client has been doing since the last contact. This step could be done via open questions, while some practitioners prefer a brief outcome measure such as a depression inventory. You and the client would agree on a measure of negative emotion, for example, and monitor that measure each session by having the client complete it at the start of the session, and then review the results in relation to the strategies tried.

In MI–CBT, you specifically ask about the change plan and any strategies the client was asked to try from the previous session. First, you elicit what the client can remember about the goals that he or she set, the steps for their implementation, and the if–then plans for addressing barriers, while continuing to reflect responses and affirm the client's ability to recall the change plan. Elicit and identify evidence of any changes big or small. Offer affirming reflections to reinforce clients for small steps and minor progress. This process is different from generic praise. As mentioned in Chapter 1, reflective statements can also be affirming when you reflect what the person said in a way that emphasizes his or her strengths or efforts. Praise is when you give your opinion on how the client is doing. Attending the current session is reason enough for a strong affirming reflection (e.g., "You persisted in coming today even though you're not sure treatment will be helpful"). Empathize with the client's inability to achieve his or her goals and the continuation of the target behaviors. Consistent with the MI style, do not yet prescribe coping strategies for the client. Rather, use the check-in to renew motivation by recalling the client's desire, ability, reasons, need, and commitment for change discussed in the previous session. Continue to reinforce change talk for managing target behaviors and session attendance with reflections and open questions to promote elaboration.

Agreeing on the Session Agenda

CBT sessions typically begin with setting a session agenda. For MI–CBT integration, we suggested beginning every session by using ATA to collaboratively set the session agenda: (1) ask for permission, (2) state planned session components, (3) elicit feedback, (4) reflect feedback, and (5) ask the client what he or she would like to add. In the case of the evaluation session(s), you might say:

> PRACTITIONER: If it's OK with you, [Ask permission] I'd like to make a plan for our session today. Usually at this point we would get more detail about

your feelings, thoughts, and behaviors, and what triggers those things. [Tell] How does that sound to you? [Ask]

CELIA: I guess that makes sense. I don't know whether I can tell you everything because I don't always remember.

PRACTITIONER: You're not sure you can remember exactly what your triggers and reactions are. [Reflect] This is something we can work through together. [Offer hope] What else would you like to add to our agenda for today? [Open question for collaborative agenda setting]

CELIA: Nothing really, but I had a big fight with my husband yesterday.

PRACTITIONER: You are struggling with your marriage and yesterday was an example. [Reflect] We can definitely talk about that and how it fits with your triggers and reactions.

Discussing the Rationale for Session Objectives

After setting the agenda, the next step is to discuss the rationale. Recall how in an MI–CBT approach, you would not *provide* the rationale but rather you would *discuss* the rationale with ATA and reflections. The goal is to elicit the client's reasons for engaging in session tasks instead of only you providing them. When discussing a rationale for a new skill, and completing an evaluation or functional assessment, it is important to elicit the client's ideas about *what* the task is as well as *why* the task is important. This latter component blends in aspects of the evoking process when engaging the client in the session agenda.

PRACTITIONER: I am wondering what you think it means to do a careful assessment of your triggers for missing medications. [Ask]

EUGENE: Well, I guess it's like when am I most likely to miss.

PRACTITIONER: Right, we want to know when, as the timing, [Reflect] but also what situations and maybe what thoughts and feelings you have when you miss. [Tell] Why do you think it would be important to carefully look at how all that fits together? [Ask]

EUGENE: I guess because then you can help me figure out what to do.

PRACTITIONER: You are hoping we can figure out how to manage these triggers. [Reflect] When we know the different things that trigger missing medications, we can come up with specific plans for situations, like your boyfriend's house, or thoughts and feelings, like when you don't want to deal with HIV or you're feeling down about yourself. [Tell] What do you think about these reasons for doing a careful assessment? [Ask]

EUGENE: Makes sense.

Collaborative Assessment

Assessments are usually conducted in a question-and-answer interview format. The danger is having the client feel interrogated and losing the spirit of MI (partnership, acceptance, compassion, evocation). The following guidelines support the MI spirit and skills while completing an evaluation with or without forms. First, while you have already addressed permission for the assessment process, it further supports autonomy to ask for permission to use any forms or other assessment tools (see Client Handouts 3.1–3.3 for assessment tools*). Allow space for refusals and alternatives. Second, reflect client statements from the previous sessions, particularly previous change talk and information that can support the assessment (e.g., initial focusing map). Third, use open questions to elicit richer information. Fourth, reflect the answer to every question. This will ensure at least a one-to-one ratio of reflections and questions, though a two-to-one ratio is preferred (Moyers, Martin, Manuel, Hendrickson, & Miller, 2005).

How do you obtain a two-to-one ratio in an assessment session? Try reflecting, then pausing. Often you will get more information following the reflection, and you can withhold your next question until the conversation stops. You may even find it helpful to count to 5 before a follow-up question, allowing the client to think and potentially elaborate without you leading the conversation. Finally, as a tip, do not ask more than three questions in a row (with reflecting in between) without a summarizing reflection. In Chapter 1 we described a summarizing reflection as a string of reflections to summarize what the client has said. Miller and Rollnick (2002) describe a summary as picking flowers and handing them back to the client in a bouquet, and thus it can be used to pull together parts of the assessment and present them in a way that suggests the next steps of case formulation and treatment planning.

PRACTITIONER: Tell me about a time when you recently overate.

MARY: Well, last Friday I ate way too much pizza.

PRACTITIONER: So eating too much pizza was a time when you were struggling with your weight plan. [Reflect] (*pause*)

MARY: Yeah, we try to have pizza and movie night on Fridays.

PRACTITIONER: Friday night is pizza night. [Reflect] (*pause; no client response*) Who was involved with pizza and movie night? [Open question]

---

*Client Handout 3.2 can be used to explore cause–effect relationships for a variety of behaviors. It is useful for low-probability behavior as well as assessing client perceptions of stimulus control. Additionally, it can be used as a focusing tool prior to conducting more complex functional assessments.

Client Handout 3.3 can be used to explore interrelationships between the factors that trigger and maintain unwanted behavior. It can also be used as a focusing tool prior to conducting more complex functional assessments, particularly with clients who are aided by visual guides.

MARY: My mom and brother. She always buys two pizzas.

PRACTITIONER: So one of your triggers is your Friday night routine. You watch a movie with your family and eat pizza, and your mom always buys a lot of pizza, which is tempting for you. [Summarize]

You can continue this process to explore other triggers. Make sure to assess antecedents for positive behaviors (i.e., situations, strategies, and social support when the client is most likely to change the target behavior) such as taking medications, avoiding drinking, or feeling less depressed. Feel free to suggest other triggers you think may be involved or that you have noticed in other clients. You offer these suggestions using ATA. Consider offering a menu of options so that you are not directing the client toward certain triggers but instead support the client's autonomy to choose what triggers are most salient. Reflections about omissions (Resnicow & McMaster, 2012) can be helpful when the client is giving limited information. Here you reflect on what the client has obviously not mentioned: "I noticed you have not mentioned the arguments with your wife and how that affects your drinking. I am curious why you have not mentioned it as we talk about triggers." However, be prepared to step back if the response is continued avoidance or discord (e.g., "It's not a problem for me" or "I don't want to talk about that"). Finally, if information obtained during the assessment process is too limited to adequately focus on a case conceptualization and treatment plan, consider self-monitoring activities (next chapter) to enhance the evaluation. (See Table 3.1 for collaborative assessment guidelines.)

TIP for Engaging in the Evaluation: Typical Day Exercise

The Typical Day Exercise (Rollnick et al., 2008) allows you to obtain information in an open-ended way when the client may be struggling to identify triggers independently. You ask the client to walk through the activities, interactions, and associated feelings he or she experiences in a typical day. For example, you might ask, "Think about yesterday and take me through it. Just tell me what happened, and, if you want, tell me how you felt about things." In using the Typical Day Exercise it may be helpful to inquire about a weekday, as well as a weekend day, because behavioral routines and patterns of distress can significantly differ from one to the other. Include MI strategies of asking permission and balancing reflections and questions.

PRACTITIONER: We have been talking about how strongly anxiety has been affecting you. It seems like it is your most pressing concern. [Reflect]

SAM: Absolutely, I am pretty anxious whenever I am around people or think about being around people.

TABLE 3.1. Collaborative Assessment Guidelines

1. *Ask permission to use any forms or other tools.*

   "I have a form that is helpful to use when trying to understand situations like yours that can have many causes. It has some questions on it that will help us to narrow down what has been going on for the past few months. Would it be OK if I use it to help guide us?"

2. *Reflect client statements from previous sessions—particularly change talk and information that can support the assessment.*

   "You mentioned in our first meeting that you need to lose weight if you're going to be comfortable hanging out outside with your friends in the summer. Tell me what you think you'd have to do to reach your goal."

3. *Use open questions.*

   "What is usually happening when you take your medications on time?"

4. *Reflect the answer to every question—striving for a minimum one-to-one ratio of reflections and questions.*

   "You take your medication more often when you don't spend the night at your boyfriend's place."

   - *Pause for approximately 5 seconds before asking a follow-up question.*
     "Why do you think that happens?"

   - *Do not ask more than three questions without a summarizing reflection.*
     "When you have a regular sleep schedule, you're at home in the morning, and you have a 'This is what I have to do, no excuses' attitude—that is when you're most likely to take your medication on time each day."

5. *Expand limited responses with MI strategies.*

   - *Ask–Tell–Ask.*
     "What do you know about the kinds of challenges people usually have with social anxiety? [Pause for client response.] Right, eating in front of people and public speaking are common sources of social anxiety. I know of a couple of others too, if you'd be interested in hearing them. [Reflect client response.] Some people find it difficult to make eye contact with others, to go to parties, to talk to an authority figure such as a supervisor, or to go on a date. How do those match with situations that make you anxious?"

   - *Menu of options.*
     "You mentioned that you deal with your anxiety by drinking alcohol or by avoiding situations in which you would have to talk in front of the class. Which of those would you like to talk about first, or maybe there is something else on your mind that is your number one priority?"

   - *Omission reflections.*
     "I noticed that, although you've mentioned how your husband reacts, you haven't mentioned how your daughter reacts when you are feeling irritable."

   - *Self-monitoring before next session.*
     "To add to what we've talked about today, I'm wondering what your thoughts are about keeping track of the days and times when you find yourself worrying about your family's safety or your own. [Reflect client response.] Some people find that also writing down what has been going on when they start worrying really adds to their understanding of what is making them worry. That would help me to do a better job of helping you too. What are your thoughts about doing that?"

PRACTITIONER: People are the main source of your anxiety. [Reflect] Sorry to hear how distressing that is. [Express empathy] In order to understand the anxiety a little better, would it be possible for you to walk me through a typical day and I will ask you about your anxiety at those times? [Ask permission]

SAM: Sure. Usually I wake up around 10, and eat breakfast in my room.

PRACTITIONER: Breakfast at 10. [Reflect] What is your anxiety on the scale we have been using—from 1 to 100?

SAM: About a 5.

PRACTITIONER: So pretty relaxed. [Reflect] OK, then what? [Open question]

SAM. Then if I have a morning class, I have to start to get ready.

PRACTITIONER: Getting ready for class is next. [Reflect] What is your anxiety like at that point? [Open question]

SAM: Well, it starts to increase a bit as it gets closer to the time I need to leave the house.

Focusing

In traditional CBT, a cognitive conceptualization provides the framework for understanding the client in terms of the cognitive model (situation → automatic thought → reaction/outcome → automatic thought). In other variants of CBT (brief or more behavioral), the focus is on triggers (who, when, what, where) that lead to the target problem or that help to avoid the target problem. These can include automatic thoughts and beliefs, but may be much broader. Regardless of the approach, the goal is the same: to collaboratively determine the links between thoughts, feelings, behaviors, and situations or other triggers that form a cycle, maintain the problem, but can lead to intervention targets. In the previous chapter, therapist and client were focusing on target behaviors or symptoms. Now they focus on intervention targets and tasks to guide the development of a treatment plan.

This process can be thought of as moving from the *why* to the *how* (Resnicow, McMaster, & Rollnick, 2012). So far we have mostly been discussing why to change and why to engage in CBT. If you are not clear about the client's "why" to change, consider returning to strategies delineated in the previous chapter. As long as you are hearing some change talk about why the client wants to change even in the midst of lingering ambivalence, then elaborating on *how* to change is warranted. In MI–CBT you collaboratively explore how to change by integrating client knowledge and preferences with your knowledge of the evidence, which includes not only research findings but also published guidelines and clinical experience (Stetler, Damschroder, Helfrich, & Hagedorn, 2011). This can be done using ATA (asking what the client knows about potential interventions for a trigger, telling what you know might work, and then asking for feedback) or with action reflections as described below.

Action Reflections

Before jumping in with advice, even in an MI-consistent way using ATA, try an action reflection (Resnicow et al., 2012). This occurs where you embed a possible future action or intervention strategy into the reflection (e.g., "You said a diet isn't going to work, so it might have to be more like a meal plan"). ATA is providing new advice from the practitioner, whereas an action reflection uses what the client has said to introduce new ideas or potential evidence-based intervention strategies. Because an action reflection is still considered a reflection of the client's perspective, it does not require permission as in ATA.

> An action reflection uses what the client has said to introduce new ideas or potential evidence-based intervention strategies.

Action reflections can be thought of as falling into three subtypes: behavioral suggestion, cognitive suggestion, and behavior exclusion. In an action reflection with a behavioral suggestion you reflect a client barrier and reframe it as an action statement. Carl is concerned about alcohol cravings. You reflect that and then say, for example, "Working on skills to manage cravings is something that could help you stay sober during probation." For Mary, who notes that nothing feels pleasurable any more, you might say, "Remembering what activities used to make you happy might help with figuring out how to bring that feeling back into your life."

A cognitive suggestion follows a similar structure but embeds a solution around thoughts instead of behaviors: "You feel like you can't do anything right and then you give up, so figuring out how to keep going when these thoughts come up might be helpful." If considering a third-wave CBT approach, you could say, "You have tried to change thoughts in the past, so an approach that includes accepting thoughts but changing behavior might work better for you."

Sometimes client statements suggest intervention strategies that are likely not effective, and an action reflection that suggests behavioral exclusion is warranted. A generic behavioral exclusion action reflection uses the following format: "It seems as though X hasn't worked, so we should cross that off the list." For example, Mary is constantly frustrated because her mother harps on her to lose weight. "From what you have said, using your mother to remind you might not work if it's nagging." You may also use this type of action reflection to communicate that you are listening carefully to interventions that the client does not want to consider. Eugene smokes marijuana on occasion and does not think this practice interferes with his medication adherence; an action reflection could be "You don't think marijuana use affects how you take your medications, so we won't focus on that right now." In this way, you communicate that you are listening carefully to the client's preferences and you avoid client discord that often sounds like "Yeah, but . . . " in response to your suggestions. Although action reflections are described here as part of the case formulation, you can use this strategy throughout your initial and subsequent sessions to ensure that intervention targets are closely tied to the client's experience and that the client experiences the intervention plan as his or her own and not just your ideas.

> **TIP for Focusing the Evaluation:**
> **Improving Your Action Reflections**
>
> Because action reflections embed suggestions or advice in a reflection, they help avoid the "righting reflex," the temptation to correct things that are perceived as wrong. As noted earlier, this reflex communicates a lack of support for client autonomy and often results in reduced collaboration. There are several ways to further avoid this situation and reduce the likelihood of discord or increased sustain talk—for example, "That will never work"; "Yeah, but I really don't want to work on that right now." First, your tone should be casual and underselling—for example, "I'm not sure, but maybe this could work"; "If there was a way to get some support without nagging, then you *might* be able to have your wife help you." Second, support autonomy by emphasizing the word "you" ("Based on what *you* said . . . "). Third, keep the advice or suggestion more general (e.g., "figuring out how your husband can help" vs. the more specific "having your husband come to sessions") or present a menu of options ("You think your husband could be more helpful, and you might consider having him give you reminders, plan outings, or maybe come to sessions down the road").

Summarizing

When you and the client have focused enough to move on to a treatment plan, it is time to transition to evoking motivation for intervention targets and then developing specifics of the plan. In CBT, this transition would include sharing of the case formulation in terms of a diagnosis and education about the cognitive-behavioral model (Beck, 2011) or presentation of a problem statement that includes symptoms, triggers, and the impact on the client's life (Papworth, Marrinan, Martin, Keegan, & Chaddock, 2013). In MI–CBT, determining an official diagnosis is unnecessary as long as the focus is specific enough to match intervention targets to evidence-based treatment strategies. That is, you do not need to use a diagnosis of "major depression" if you can guide the client to identify his or her symptoms and triggers. A problem statement can avoid the diagnosis and focus on symptoms and triggers, but it does not include potential intervention targets and misses an opportunity to increase hope and optimism. For some clients, however, knowing their diagnosis can be helpful in that it helps to normalize their problem and indicates that effective treatments are available.

In MI–CBT, consider using a summarizing reflection to transition to evoking motivation for intervention targets and developing the specifics of the treatment plan. The summary would capture elements of the assessment and the formulation, ending with a key question about what the client would like to do with this information—for example:

> "We have talked about a lot of things that get in the way of your weight loss. You get depressed about it, which makes you lie around more and avoid exercise. You eat more when you're depressed, and the fun your family has usually includes unhealthy foods. You are thinking about how to find an exercise that is fun and burns calories, how to manage the depressed thoughts and feelings, and how to get your family to be more supportive without nagging."

This summary can be followed with a key question about next steps in the treatment plan: "What do you see as the next step?" Alternatively, you can end with a question to elicit change talk, as described in the following section: "How do you think things could be better if you found an activity you enjoyed?"

You may consider recording the options for intervention targets on a form or diagram (Miller, 2004). Some prefer to record information throughout the session, but we often find that this can distract from the processes. Instead, you may prefer to fill out a form or diagram when summarizing (see Client Handout 3.4*). In the example in Figure 3.1, Mary's difficulty with eating and physical activity choices are the target behaviors and the factors triggering these choices are recorded in the boxes. A treatment plan subsequently addresses the primary triggers. Some practitioners may find it helpful to use separate diagrams for facilitators and barriers, while others may prefer to put everything on one diagram.

Evoking

In the previous chapter, we discussed how to elicit and reinforce change talk, which refers to desire, ability, reasons, need, and commitment to changing the target behaviors. Now the emphasis of evoking is not so much on whether to change as on

---

*Client Handout 3.4 can be used to summarize cause–effect relationships for a variety of behaviors. It can also be used for focusing and planning, particularly with clients who are aided by visual guides.

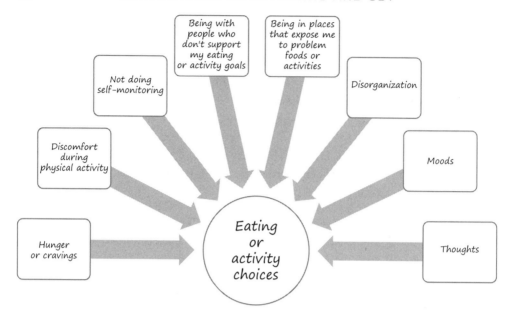

FIGURE 3.1. Example of focusing: Summarizing Mary's intervention targets.

how to change, though ambivalence about behavior change may still arise and need exploration. Thus, the change talk we are looking for here sounds like desire, ability, reasons, need, and commitment about how to change. Examples include "I want to learn how to refuse sugary foods" or "I need to figure out how to make myself do more activities." The strategies described in the previous chapter, such as open questions to elicit change talk, would now ask about potential treatment components. You can refer to any forms utilized in the engaging and focusing stage and elicit change talk about potential intervention targets: "Why would you want to consider scheduling activities that used to be fun?" or "What's the best thing that could happen if you learned to manage your thoughts about avoiding your diagnosis?" It is critical not to skip over this process and assume that a shared case formulation and treatment plan are sufficient to build motivation for treatment participation.

Personalized Feedback

There is some evidence to suggest that MI combined with feedback of assessment results has a stronger effect on evoking motivation for change than MI without feedback (Walters, Vader, Harris, Field, & Jouriles, 2009). Personalized feedback involves presenting factual information with the goals of increasing concern about the target behavior and awareness of its triggers to build motivation for the treatment plan. The information comes from either objective assessments (e.g., lab results, urine screens) or from the client's self-report. Utilizing ATA, you will provide only facts, without judgment or analysis of the results. You will elicit the client's interpretation of feedback in terms of the case conceptualization, building motivation for the treatment plan. Assessments useful for feedback include level of target behavior, problems or consequences of target behavior including objective health information, temptations or triggers for target behavior, and treatment goals (e.g., What I Want from Treatment questionnaire; *https://casaa.unm.edu/ inst/What%20I%20Want%20From%20Treatment.pdf*).

PRACTITIONER: Before we move on, I was wondering what you would like to know about the questionnaires you completed? [Ask]

CARL: I was wondering what it was all about. I really don't drink that much.

PRACTITIONER: You don't think you drink excessively. [Reflect] Based on your report, if you add up the days you drank, you said you drank 20 out of the last 30 days for a total of 100 drinks. [Tell] How does that fit with your thoughts about your drinking? [Ask]

CARL: Well, I guess I did not realize I was drinking that much almost every day.

PRACTITIONER: You are wondering if you are drinking more than you realized. [Reflect change talk]

CARL: Yeah, I'm OK with drinking, but I don't want to be a daily drinker.

PRACTITIONER: Being a daily drinker does not fit with who you want to be. [Reflect change talk] You also reported that you feel least confident about controlling your drinking when you are in social situations and when you have strong cravings. [Tell] How should we address that in your treatment plan? [Ask]

CARL: I will definitely need help with those things if I am going to survive probation. [Change talk]

PRACTITIONER: You're thinking the treatment plan should include skills to manage social events and how to handle cravings. [Reflect change talk in terms of treatment plan]

The client may question results from the objective assessment or the self-report questionnaires (e.g., "This can't be right—these questions are stupid anyway"). As with all forms of sustain talk, you simply reflect these statements or use other strategies described in the previous chapter and further explore how the client sees the situation—for example: "OK, so as you see it, the assessment was not right. How much do you think you have been drinking, and what do you see as the biggest barriers to reaching your goal?" In this way, you emphasize your respect for the client's point of view while continuing to build motivation for the treatment plan. (See Table 3.2 for additional strategies to provide feedback.)

TABLE 3.2. Tips for Feedback Discussions

1. *Introduce the use of personalized feedback.*
   "You recall I mentioned that we were going to look at some of the results of all those tests and assessments you completed before you entered the study."

2. *Affirm the client for participation and emphasize autonomy.*
   "I know that there were a lot of them, and we appreciate the time you took. If it's OK with you, I'd like to share that information and you can let me know how useful it is to you."

3. *Introduce feedback data in context.*
   "This is a summary of the results of the assessments you completed. You gave us some really important information about what things have been like for you and what's been happening in your life. Would you mind if I share with you what jumps out at me in this information?"

4. *Remind the client of the specific measure that gave a particular result and explain what the instrument was attempting to assess* (self-report or assessor administered; types of questions [e.g., multiple choice, yes/no]; examples of questions asked; assessing problems associated with drug use; how much medications are missed; triggers for depressed mood).

5. *Give an overview of the scheme of measurement.*
   "This score tells you. . . ."

6. *Point out the score or result.*
   "As you can see here, your score added up to 43. . . ."
   but nonjudgmentally and accept disagreement. Roll with resistance. *Elicit the client's reaction.*
   "How does this sound to you? How well does this fit with what your life has been like?"
   and provide relevant information with permission.
   "If you would like, I have some information about how getting chlamydia affects your HIV status."

7. *Reflect and summarize the client's overt reactions. Double-sided reflections are often helpful here.*
   "Not all of this information feels like it fits. On the other hand, some of it is leading you to think that you have been strongly affected by the missing medications, like when you were in the hospital."

8. *Reflect the client's nonverbal reactions.*
   "I noticed that when I said that, your eyes got wide for a moment. What was it like for you to hear how much marijuana you smoked in the last month?" or "I noticed that when I said that your mood was in the moderately depressed range, it seemed to really strike a chord."

9. *Make a transition to the next result.*
   "So far, we've been focusing on viral load; this next piece of information may tell us something important about how your substance use fits into the picture." or "We have been focusing on how avoiding situations you fear can maintain one's anxiety; now I want to ask about what happens when you are forced to be in these types of situations."

10. *Give intermediate summaries.*
    "Not only has being depressed gotten in the way of taking care of things that are important to you, but getting high on a daily basis led you to think about giving up."

11. *Provide a final summary.*
    "So the assessments you completed suggested that you miss your medications about half the time, your viral load is high, and you often miss a dose when you use alcohol. At the same time, you've got some mixed feelings about quitting alcohol though you're interested in cutting back before you take your medications. Is that about right?"

12. *Elicit change talk by asking how these behaviors fit with broad life goals.*
    "One of the things you've come back to a couple of times is how important it is to for you to be more active for your children. What are your thoughts about this now after looking together at these results?"

Planning

If you have followed the guidelines for the other three processes, you already have been doing bits of planning throughout the evaluation session(s) by assessing triggers, focusing on intervention targets, and building motivation to address them. In the planning process, you further specify the plan for treatment as well the plan for the next session. The following elements should be covered in the planning process of the evaluation component of treatment.

Asking for Permission

First, ask for permission to engage in a treatment plan. While the client may realize that every session will end with a change plan as in the first session, he or she may not be prepared for a full treatment plan, particularly not a written plan as typically done in research trials and for insurance purposes. At this point in the evaluation session, if the rest of the processes have gone well, the client is often ready to engage in this task. However, if necessary, discuss the rationale using ATA and respond to discord or increased sustain talk as discussed in the last chapter.

Reviewing and Prioritizing Intervention Targets

Next, you review the identified target areas and any forms completed using a summarizing reflection and asking for elaboration if any are missed at this point. Then, you and your client prioritize those components, once again guiding the client to consider his or her own preferences as well as any evidence suggesting priorities.

> PRACTITIONER: We have talked about your triggers and you think it would be helpful if you understood how your thoughts link to your symptoms. Increasing your activity and improving your relationship with your husband are also things we would work on together in the next sessions. What else would you like to add as a priority target area? [Ask]
>
> CELIA: Well, I still would like to go back to school.
>
> PRACTITIONER: School is a priority for you. We can add that to your plan. [Tell] From the perspective of a CBT treatment, this might fall in the same category as increasing your activity level because it would involve getting up, going out, doing homework for school, and interacting with others. How does that sound? [Ask]
>
> CELIA: I guess that sounds good.
>
> PRACTITIONER. OK, well let's together determine which goals we should work on in the weeks ahead. Let's discuss which ones are most important to

you, and I can offer information about which ones seem to help other clients with similar goals.

CELIA: I want to work on my marriage, but I know that the other things like the worries and low energy are really keeping me stuck.

PRACTITIONER: Your marriage is a priority, but you think that you might need to work on other things first so that you are more successful when you tackle the relationship issues. Managing worries and increasing activities are both important. It's up to you what you want to work on first. We will get to both for sure.

CELIA: I guess the worries and getting lost in my thoughts first. I am not sure I'm ready to do any new activities right now even if it is something fun.

Collaboratively Specifying the Treatment Plan

The third component is the specification of a treatment plan in order of priority based on the previous discussion (see Client Handout 3.5*). The plan is preferably written with permission from the client. A nice strategy to support autonomy is to offer the client the choice of writing it down him- or herself or to have you write it down for him or her. Not all items on the treatment plan must be addressed in sessions, and some may be addressed by the client on his or her own (e.g., making an appointment with a physician, spending more time with daughter) or with referrals (e.g., support group). For each target, you and the client collaboratively specify the problem to be addressed, the broad goals and the specific objectives, and the planned intervention strategies (see Figure 3.2 for a treatment plan example). You use open questions, reflections, and ATA to integrate client knowledge and preferences with the information you have about evidence-based treatments (e.g., self-monitoring, skills training, activity scheduling).

If the evidence is not clear on which intervention strategy should target a particular trigger (e.g., cognitive restructuring, acceptance-based approaches, or behavioral experiments), options can be presented and prioritized with the client. If your treatment uses a module format, specific modules and their order of delivery may similarly be chosen collaboratively. If you have not elicited and discussed with the client intervention goals and strategies that you think might be critical, it is OK to bring them up with ATA and a menu of options: "Some people have said that not wanting anyone to know their diagnosis gets in the way of taking HIV medication sometimes. What do you think about that as a potential trigger?"

In CBT for anxiety, the practitioner and client face the difficult task of the treatment itself, namely, exposure sessions, where the client does the very thing that is so anxiety-provoking and the cause of tremendous distress. Once

---

*Client Handout 3.5 can be used to address presenting problems and other issues that arise during assessment and/or treatment. It is primarily a planning tool, but may aid the focusing process.

Target Behavior/ Symptom/Concern	Goals and Objectives	Treatment Plan
1. Alcohol use	a. Complete probation with no positive alcohol screens	Self-monitoring of alcohol Managing cravings Refusal skills
2. Feeling depressed	a. Don't drink when feeling sad (above 20 on 0–100 rating scale) b. Do at least one pleasurable activity every day	2a. Self-monitoring of mood 2b. Activity scheduling
3. Marital conflict	a. Improve relationship with wife	Communication skills Managing thoughts— all-or-nothing thinking Anger management

Three reasons why this plan is important to me:

1. *I don't want to go to prison.*

2. *I want to stay married to my wife.*

3. *I want to save money by not having to be in treatment anymore.*

FIGURE 3.2. Carl's sample treatment plan.

the practitioner has gained an understanding of the difficulties, and has developed a working case conceptualization, he or she must explain how the treatment will work and help the client understand that engaging in this treatment should reduce the client's distress in the long run. Clients may be turned off to treatment just thinking about having to face items high on their fear hierarchies for exposures.

SAM: Yikes, as we are discussing this, I am not quite sure how you would expect me to do the kinds of things you are talking about.

PRACTITIONER: Yes, what I am talking about can seem hard, especially the situations that are higher on your fear hierarchy. [Reflect]

SAM: Exactly. Like I just cannot even imagine taking a class where participation is part of the grade and where I need to do a presentation.

PRACTITIONER: You would be pretty anxious considering doing that. [Reflect]

SAM: Even talking about it now makes me start to sweat.

PRACTITIONER: OK. So it is really up to you whether you are ready to tackle these fears. [Emphasize personal choice] What about starting with some of the items that are much lower on the list, and waiting to tackle those higher on the list until you feel more ready?

SAM: That could work.

PRACTITIONER: You see how gradually exposing yourself to these fears might help. [Reflect] Where would you like to start on this list? [Emphasize personal choice]

SAM: What about this one, having a meal in the student center instead of in my room?

Consolidating Commitment to the Treatment Plan

Finally, you begin guiding the client to consolidate commitment with a summarizing reflection, recapitulating change talk for *why* to change and *how* to change and incorporating next steps in the treatment plan—for example:

> "Eugene, we have talked about why you want to take your medications—to maintain your health and your independence. You see the importance of keeping track of how often you miss taking your meds, improving your planning when you spend the night at your boyfriend's, and managing the negative thoughts you have about your status. You want to start with tracking how often you miss your meds and making plans for sleepovers. What have I missed?"

If the client responds with additions or changes, reflect these and amend the treatment plan if necessary. Now ask for a verbal commitment to move forward on the plan. Some examples include: "What do you think about your commitment to this plan?" or "Why do you feel this plan is something you must do?" Always reinforce commitment language with reflections or by asking for elaboration. Consider a commitment ruler as described in the previous chapter.

> Ask for a verbal commitment to move forward on the plan.

Planning for the Next Session

In MI–CBT you end every session with a specific change plan for the next week that includes a goal for the week, specific steps to achieve that goal, and the development of if–then plans to address barriers to goal achievement. At this point in treatment, the client may choose the goal of reducing the problem behavior, but this goal may be premature if the client does not have the skills to do so. Alternatives could be to make small behavioral changes ("I am going to stop drinking hard liquor"; "I am going to try to walk the dog tomorrow"). However, in MI–CBT we begin to orient the client to the concept of between-session practice at the onset of treatment. These assignments can be thought of as part of the specific steps of the change plan, and at this point can include reviewing the treatment plan, obtaining additional information (e.g., record problem behaviors, symptoms, or situations; interview family members), preparing for the next intervention strategy (e.g., make a list of possible pleasurable activities), or completing a self-help intervention (e.g., attending a support group, reading a relevant chapter, or practicing 5 minutes of meditation). As with any treatment task, discuss the assignment and the rationale using ATA (see section above), eliciting as much as you can from the client before providing information. At the end of relevant chapters is a change plan form for the tasks associated with that chapter (see Client Handout 3.6). Celia's completed Change Plan form specific to an assessment session is shown in Figure 3.3. Chapter 7 on homework has further discussion of how to increase motivation

---

My Plan to Get Started

Changes I would like to make:

Understand how my thoughts relate to my symptoms

Increase my activity

Improve my relationship with my husband

These changes are important to me because:

I do not want my thoughts and worries to control me

I want to be able to drive without worrying that something bad will happen

I want to go back to school

My marriage is important to me

I want to have energy again

I plan to take these steps to get started (what, where, when, how):

Make a list of the things that trigger my worries before my next session. I will do this

on Wednesday when the kids don't have any activities.

Ask my husband to drive me to my next session if I don't think I can do it myself

(Query about session attendance if not spontaneously provided.)

IF this gets in the way	THEN try this
I forget to make a list of triggers	Put a reminder in my phone calendar
	before I have a chance to forget
I can't think of my triggers	Ask my husband and daughter to help me
I need my husband to drive me to	Ask my sister, or my neighbor to be my
my next session, but he can't	back-up ride

FIGURE 3.3. Celia's Change Plan.

for assignments and how to manage discord and sustain talk when homework is missed, though a separate change plan for this chapter is not applicable as assignments are included in each chapter's change plan.

PRACTITIONER: Now that we have discussed various situations that make you anxious, I wanted to bring up the idea of making progress outside of the sessions. Do you have a sense of what I am talking about here?

SAM: Well, I think so. I had heard that CBT involved "homework."

PRACTITIONER: Well, basically it does. I like to call it "between-session practice" because "homework" sounds a bit like school, but regardless, can we discuss this a bit more?

SAM: Sure. So, what are you going to assign then?

PRACTITIONER: I am glad you asked it like that, because this issue of "homework" sounds more like it is an assignment from me. Instead, we should, together, agree on what kinds of next steps you could try outside of the sessions to keep progress going when we are not together in the office. How do you think that is different?

SAM: Well, you are saying that I have a say in what the homework is.

PRACTITIONER: Even more than that, you not only have a say, but we should talk together about what it is that we both think will be best for you.

SAM: OK, I see.

PRACTITIONER: Do you have a sense of why this might be important in treating anxiety?

SAM: Well, for one thing, I think what you are going to ask me to do will be hard.

PRACTITIONER: Well, it might be. But what if we are really careful to make sure that it is not me asking you to do things per se, but instead, us coming up with good next steps together that are not so hard that you won't or can't do them, but not so easy that they are not doing much for your progress?

SAM: Well, that sounds a lot better.

MI–CBT Dilemmas

An ongoing dilemma is how to proceed if ambivalence is still present. This problem might be most obvious when the client does not commit to the treatment plan, but it can also be noticed throughout the other processes with sustain talk and discord. You might choose to continue with MI-only following the guidelines in the previous chapter, or you might decide to forge ahead with CBT and see what happens. We believe that there is always some ambivalence about change, but that CBT should proceed if you can get some agreement on a treatment plan. An option is to see if the client will commit to trying just one or two treatment strategies (e.g., self-monitoring, physical activity) before deciding to commit to the whole plan. Sometimes a time limit will help the client to commit, trying one intervention strategy for a few weeks before deciding to continue. If the client absolutely refuses to engage in CBT, we believe that a few MI sessions can tip the scale of ambivalence in favor of change, but most studies of MI by itself have not included more than a few sessions (Lundahl & Burke, 2009). Thus, we recommend an approach from motivational enhancement therapy (Miller, Zweben, & DiClemente, 1994), where you see the client for a few initial motivational sessions and then follow-up in a month and see if the client is ready to engage in CBT or would prefer to continue on his or her own.

Another dilemma occurs when the client's preferences for the treatment plan run counter to what you know of the evidence. Sometimes the client's ideas can simply be added to the plan, for example, if the client believes that nutritional supplements will help with depression. Other times the client's goal clearly contradicts the evidence. For example, the client prefers a goal of alcohol moderation, but the evidence suggests that an abstinence approach would be more likely to succeed. We believe that you present the information with ATA but ultimately go with the client's preference. You and the client can consider the client's choice of goal as a hypothesis, and the two of you will gather evidence to see if the plan is effective over a set time frame (long enough to test the hypothesis but not so long as to result in treatment failure). You can consider other options if desired outcomes are not achieved. Even if you cannot ethically convey optimism, you can still convey hope that the client's preference will work, building the alliance so that your advice will be considered in the future if the client is still struggling. If the client's preference is contraindicated (e.g., "I only want to take my HIV medications every other day"), then ethically you must provide this information with ATA and cannot follow this approach.

Finally, you may come across a client who refuses to consider homework. You can try to elicit the rationale for homework and the client's ideas for homework that seem relevant, palatable, and feasible. CBT approaches stress the idea that much of the progress occurs between sessions, and that homework is the vehicle for that progress. If the client absolutely refuses to do homework, and you believe that CBT cannot proceed without homework, you can explain that you cannot do CBT until the client is ready for homework and move on to the motivational enhancement therapy approach described above. Alternatively, you can decide to provide some components of CBT, explaining that they may not work as efficiently without homework but you are certainly willing to work with the client and try. There is no right answer here. We believe that any treatment is better than no treatment at all as long as you don't undermine the client's belief in the treatment's efficacy because outcomes may not be strong without all treatment components.

Functional Assessment Three Ways

Traditional functional assessment follows a question-and-answer interview format. Two alternatives maintain MI spirit and skills and build motivation for the treatment plan. One way is to follow each open question with a reflection, and summarize after every three questions. Even better is reflecting the information you have already obtained in previous conversations and integrating them into a functional assessment using pauses and open questions to guide the client to elaborate.

ACTIVITY GOAL: In this activity you will practice how to complete a functional assessment in an MI–CBT integrated approach.

ACTIVITY INSTRUCTIONS: Consider the following five questions excerpted from a functional assessment from a weight loss trial, specifically targeting overeating. Note that you can ask the same questions for eating less or following the meal plan. Fill in the blanks for the second two versions.

Version 1: Interview

1. *People:* Are there certain people usually around when you eat large portions of food, like filling up the whole plate, going back for seconds, or having a snack that you shouldn't have if you want to keep your calories down? For example, are you more likely to overeat with particular friends, classmates, siblings, or family members?

   MARY: I definitely eat more with my family. I don't like to eat too much around my friends except when we go out to eat on special occasions.

2. *Places*: Are there any places that make it harder to eat less? For example, at school, at church, at a relative's or neighbor's home, or at a fast-food restaurant?

   MARY: When I go out to eat with my friends, we usually go to McDonalds or the corner store. Then I feel more out of control.

3. *Emotions*: Do you notice any particular emotion, mood, or feeling that you are in when you eat more than you should? These could include being sad, angry, tired, or bored.

   MARY: I eat more when I feel sad and bored. Like when I get depressed about my weight and I don't feel like moving. Then I'm bored because I have nothing to do.

4. *Times*: Are there times of day or days of the week when it is harder to eat less? For example, is overeating more likely to happen at night, during lunch at school, when your mother is at work, or when you're watching TV?

   MARY: After school if we hang out, then Friday night pizza and movie night with my mom.

5. *Thoughts*: Are there certain thoughts that go through your head when you overeat? For example, hopelessness, thoughts of rejection?

> MARY: I don't know. Maybe when I feel out of control, it's like I can't stop and then I'm like what's wrong with me.

Version 2: Ask–Reflect–Ask–Reflect and Summarize

First, change the question to an open-ended one. Then, add a reflection in between each question and summarize after three questions. Your reflection can be a simple paraphrase or can be more complex as in an action reflection. We demonstrate with the first question.

1. *People:* Are certain people usually around when you eat large portions of food, like filling up the whole plate, going back for seconds, or having a snack that you shouldn't have if you want to keep your calories down? For example, are you more likely to overeat with particular friends, classmates, siblings, or family members?

> PRACTITIONER [Open question]: What people are usually around when you eat large portions of food, like friends or family?

> MARY: I definitely eat more with my family. I don't like to eat too much around my friends except when we go out to eat on special occasions.

> PRACTITIONER [Reflect]: Family members are the main people you overeat with and friends only on special occasions.

> ACTION REFLECTION: Family members are the main people you overeat with and friends only on special occasions, so figuring out how to help people support you might be useful.

2. *Places*: Are there any places that make it harder to eat less? For example, at school, at church, at a relative's or neighbor's home, or at a fast-food restaurant?

> PRACTITIONER [Open question]: _____

> _____

> MARY: When I go out to eat with my friends, we usually go to McDonalds or the corner store. Then I feel more out of control.

> PRACTITIONER [Reflect]: _____

> _____

3. *Emotions*: Do you notice any particular emotion, mood, or feeling that you are in when you eat more than you should? These could include being sad, angry, tired, or bored.

> PRACTITIONER [Open question]: _____

> _____

> MARY: I eat more when I feel sad and bored. Like when I get depressed about my weight and I don't feel like moving. Then I'm bored because I have nothing to do.

PRACTITIONER [Reflect]: _____

_____

SUMMARY: So far, you know that you eat more with family members in general and you overeat more with your friends when you go to McDonald's or the corner store. When this happens you feel out of control and like there is something wrong with you.

4. *Times*: Are there times of day or days of the week when it is harder to eat less? For example, is overeating more likely to happen at night, during lunch at school, when your mother is at work, or when you're watching TV?

PRACTITIONER [Open question]: _____

_____

MARY: After school if we hang out, then Friday night pizza and movie night with my mom.

PRACTITIONER [Reflect]: _____

_____

5. Thoughts: Are there certain thoughts that go through your head when you overeat? For example, feeling hopeless, rejected, or unloved?

PRACTITIONER [Open question]: _____

_____

MARY: I don't know. Maybe when I feel out of control, it's like I can't stop and then I'm like what's wrong with me.

PRACTITIONER [Reflect]: _____

_____

OVERALL SUMMARY: _____

Version 3

See what answers you can glean from the conversation without asking any questions.

PRACTITIONER: Mary, in order for us to figure out the best plan, it would be helpful to find out more about the people, places, thoughts, and moods that trigger eating too much.

MARY: Well, I definitely eat more when I'm feeling down. Like hopeless about everything. And then my mom comes in with pizza for our movie night, and I just go nuts.

PRACTITIONER: You eat more with your family, especially on movie nights when you're feeling hopeless and overwhelmed.

MARY: Yeah. I don't really overeat with my friends unless we are going to McDonald's or something. We only do that once in a while.

What did you learn about people? _____

About places? _____

About moods? _____

About thoughts? _____

About times? _____

What questions remain? _____

_____

MI Spirit in the Evaluation

ACTIVITY GOAL: In this activity you will decide which approach feels most consistent with MI spirit.

ACTIVITY INSTRUCTIONS: Role-play each version of the functional assessment in Activity 3.1 with a partner. Rate each role play in terms of the four components of MI spirit (partnership, acceptance, compassion, evocation) using the scaling forms below. Discuss the trade-offs between MI spirit and CBT assessment goals.

Functional Assessment Version 1: Interview

Partnership						
We are working against each other (Wrestling)			We are working in partnership (Dancing)			We are in the room, but not much is happening (Standing)
1	2	3	4	5	6	7
Acceptance						
I struggle with the client's choices and/ or press the client to change (Directing)			I recognize and honor client's choices, including no change (Accepting)			I seem indifferent to client's wishes or choices (Observing)
1	2	3	4	5	6	7

Compassion						
Outcomes are more important than client needs (Detached)			I actively and subjectively promote client's needs (Empathetic)			My reaction to client's needs is influenced by emotion (Sympathetic)
1	2	3	4	5	6	7
Evocation						
I am presenting the reasons for change (Advocating)			I am drawing out the client's views on change (Guiding)			I just let the session go wherever it will (Following)
1	2	3	4	5	6	7

Functional Assessment Version 2: Ask–Reflect–Ask–Summarize

Partnership						
We are working against each other (Wrestling)			We are working in partnership (Dancing)			We are in the room, but not much is happening (Standing)
1	2	3	4	5	6	7
Acceptance						
I struggle with the client's choices and/ or press the client to change (Directing)			I recognize and honor client's choices, including no change (Accepting)			I seem indifferent to client's wishes or choices (Observing)
1	2	3	4	5	6	7
Compassion						
Outcomes are more important than client needs (Detached)			I actively and subjectively promote client's needs (Empathetic)			My reaction to client's needs is influenced by emotion (Sympathetic)
1	2	3	4	5	6	7

Evocation						
I am presenting the reasons for change (Advocating)			I am drawing out the client's views on change (Guiding)			I just let the session go wherever it will (Following)
1	2	3	4	5	6	7

Functional Assessment Version 3: Conversation

Partnership						
We are working against each other (Wrestling)			We are working in partnership (Dancing)			We are in the room, but not much is happening (Standing)
1	2	3	4	5	6	7

Acceptance						
I struggle with the client's choices and/ or press the client to change (Directing)			I recognize and honor client's choices, including no change (Accepting)			I seem indifferent to client's wishes or choices (Observing)
1	2	3	4	5	6	7

Compassion						
Outcomes are more important than client needs (Detached)			I actively and subjectively promote client's needs (Empathetic)			My reaction to client's needs is influenced by emotion (Sympathetic)
1	2	3	4	5	6	7

Evocation						
I am presenting the reasons for change (Advocating)			I am drawing out the client's views on change (Guiding)			I just let the session go wherever it will (Following)
1	2	3	4	5	6	7

Action Reflections

ACTIVITY GOAL: In this activity you will practice forming action reflections to embed intervention ideas into reflective statements.

ACTIVITY INSTRUCTIONS: For each type of action reflection, formulate your answers. See suggested responses at the end of the activity.

1. *Behavioral suggestion:* Reflect a client barrier and reframe as an action statement.

   a. Eugene tells you that he stopped taking his antiretroviral medication since he missed his last medical visit and has run out of medication. What might you say below to convey an understanding for the barrier but then also giving an action statement?

   _____

   _____

   b. Carl states that he doesn't want to be in alcohol treatment, but he doesn't want to lose his family or go to jail either. He wants everyone to stop hassling him and for things to go back to the way they were before his motor vehicle accident.

   _____

   _____

2. *Cognitive suggestion:* Reflect a client barrier and reframe as suggestion for changing thoughts.

   a. Celia worries that driving will result in injury to her family or herself. She needs to be able to drive to get to work, transport her children to and from school and sports events, and engage in other activities such as grocery shopping and attending medical and dental appointments. She feels hopeless that she can overcome her worries about safety.

   _____

   _____

   b. Mary says that she can't be successful with weight loss when all her mother does is nag her and bring junk food home for her younger brothers. She wants to lose weight before the summer, but she really doesn't think she can since her mother doesn't support her.

   _____

   _____

3. *Behavior exclusion:* Reflect a client barrier and identify a solution to be excluded.

   a. Carl has tried to cut back on his drinking at family gatherings at least twice before, but it didn't work. He wants to be successful, but he doesn't want to stop seeing his extended family. Drinking is a big part of their parties and other family gatherings.

   _____

   _____

   b. Sam has tried using "liquid courage" to overcome his social anxiety at parties on previous occasions, but he became very intoxicated and the strategy backfired. It's not something that he thinks will be effective, but he doesn't know what else to do.

   _____

   _____

Suggested Responses

1. *Behavioral suggestion:* Reflect a client barrier and reframe as an action statement.

   a. Eugene has stopped taking his antiretroviral medication since he missed his last medical visit and has run out of medication.

   If you can get to the clinic, then you can fill your prescription if you want to.

   b. Carl doesn't want to be in alcohol treatment, but he doesn't want to lose his family or go to jail either. He wants everyone to stop hassling him and for things to go back to the way they were before his motor vehicle accident.

   If you can attend treatment sessions, then you can get people off your back.

2. *Cognitive suggestion:* Reflect a client barrier and reframe as a restructured thought.

   a. Celia worries that driving will result in injury to her family or herself. She needs to be able to drive to get to work, transport her children to and from school and sports events, and engage in other activities such as grocery shopping and attending medical and dental appointments. She feels hopeless that she can overcome her worries about safety.

   Your worries about safety can be overwhelming, and figuring out a way to do the things that you need to do even when you have those thoughts would be helpful.

   b. Mary says that she can't be successful with weight loss when all her mother does is nag her and bring junk food home for her younger brothers. She wants to lose weight before the summer, but she really doesn't think she can since her mother doesn't support her.

   You feel like you're not getting any support at home, so finding a way to feel successful anyway would be an important part of what we work on together.

3. *Behavior exclusion:* Reflect a client barrier and identify a solution to be excluded.

   a. Carl has tried to cut back on his drinking at family gatherings at least twice before, but it didn't work. He wants to be successful, but he doesn't want to stop seeing his extended family. Drinking is a big part of their parties and other family gatherings.

   You've already tried cutting back on your drinking at family get-togethers and you don't want to stop seeing your family, so you'd rather focus on taking other steps first.

   b. Sam has tried using "liquid courage" to overcome his social anxiety at parties on previous occasions, but he became very intoxicated and the strategy backfired. It's not something that he thinks will be effective, but he doesn't know what else to do.

   You don't see an option that will help you to be more comfortable at parties right now, so maybe we should start with building your skills in other settings.

ACTIVITY 3.4 FOR PRACTITIONERS

Sequences: Eliciting and Supporting Change Talk for Treatment Planning

ACTIVITY GOAL: In this activity you will practice developing evoking questions to elicit change talk specifically for the treatment plan. You will then develop a reflection to further support the change talk.

ACTIVITY INSTRUCTIONS: For each of the following items, fill in the blanks, making up additional details of the case as necessary. You will practice completing each of the three components of the sequences. In the first section, you will complete one of the three components of the sequence (question to elicit change talk, client change talk, reflection of change talk). In the second section, you will use your creativity to complete two of the three components.

Item 1

- **Practitioner Strategy to Elicit Change Talk:** What do you want to happen?
- **Client Change Talk:** I want to be able to get together with my family without getting in trouble for drinking too much. I want to stay out of jail too.

- **Practitioner Reinforcement (Reflection/Question):** _____

_____

Item 2

- **Practitioner Strategy to Elicit Change Talk:** How do you think you could do that?

- **Client Change Talk:** _____
  _____

- **Practitioner Reinforcement (Reflection/Question):** Being able to leave after a couple of beers is a solution that you could see yourself using.

Item 3

- **Practitioner Strategy to Elicit Change Talk:** _____
  _____

- **Client Change Talk:** I'd be able to stay out of jail and I think my wife would stick with me if I can make this work.
- **Practitioner Reinforcement (Reflection/Question):** You can see how things might work out the way you want them to if we can find solutions that work for you.

Item 4

- **Practitioner Strategy to Elicit Change Talk:** Mary, now that we've talked about the things that you'd like your mother to change, such as the kind of food she brings in the house and how she talks to you when you eat it, what personal changes would you like to make?

- **Client Change Talk:** _____
  _____

- **Practitioner Reinforcement (Reflection/Question):** _____
  _____

Item 5

- **Practitioner Strategy to Elicit Change Talk:** _____
  _____

- **Client Change Talk:** I know that I need to eat less and try not to snack between meals. I probably have to drink more water and stay away from fast food too.

- **Practitioner Reinforcement (Reflection/Question):** _____
  _____

Item 6

- **Practitioner Strategy to Elicit Change Talk:** _____
  _____

- **Client Change Talk:** _____
  _____

- **Practitioner Reinforcement (Reflection/Question):** They are necessary changes for weight loss.

Suggested Responses:

Item 1

- **Practitioner Reinforcement (Reflection/Question):** You want to go to your family gatherings and avoid drinking too much.

Item 2

- **Client Change Talk:** Maybe I could leave after a couple of beers instead of staying the whole time.

Item 3

- **Practitioner Strategy to Elicit Change Talk:** What's the best thing that could happen if you learn to make this work?

Item 4

- **Client Change Talk:** I want to eat healthier and start working out.
- **Practitioner Reinforcement (Reflection/Question):** You have clear ideas about healthy weight management.

Item 5

- **Practitioner Strategy to Elicit Change Talk:** What do you already know about how to eat healthier?
- **Practitioner Reinforcement (Reflection/Question):** Making healthier eating choices is your top priority and you already have some ideas about how to do it.

Item 6

- **Practitioner Strategy to Elicit Change Talk:** Why is that important to you?
- **Client Change Talk:** I can't really lose weight without changing what I eat.

Functional Assessment Tool

Understanding when and why unwanted behavior occurs will help with planning to prevent it or to manage it differently. List the most frequent occurrences of
_____. Try to describe the requested information as fully as possible.

Where/ Situation	Who Is Present	Time of Day	Cravings	Thoughts	Feelings

Functional Assessment Tool Simplified

Understanding when and why unwanted behavior occurs, and what its effects are, will help with planning to prevent it or to manage it differently. In the "Triggers" column, make a list of the situations, people, places, etc., that you think leads to
_____. In the "Effects" column, write what happens when you are around a trigger.

Triggers	Effects

CBT Model Functional Assessment Tool

Understanding when and why unwanted behavior occurs will help with planning to prevent it or to manage it differently. Think about when _____ is most likely to occur. Use the graphic below to describe the most common situation, thoughts, emotions, physical symptoms, and behavior or activity level changes that you have when the unwanted behavior occurs.

These factors are related to one another. Changing one (i.e., thoughts) can change the others, which can change the unwanted behavior.

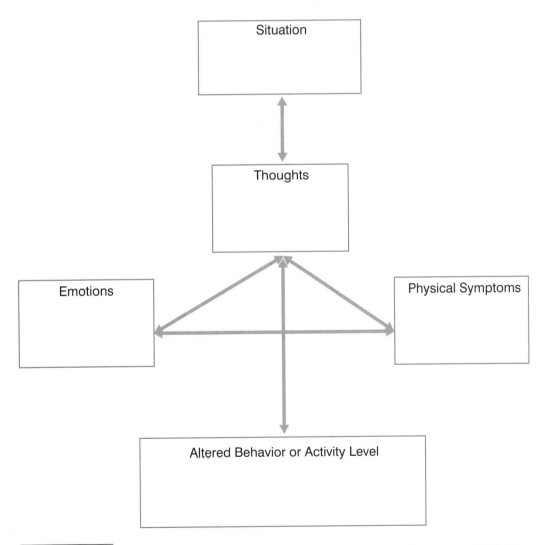

Summary of Assessment

Complete this form with your practitioner after you have finished assessing the triggers of your unwanted behavior. Write the unwanted behavior in the circle and write the triggers in the squares. Then, number the top four triggers—the ones that *most* contribute to the unwanted behavior (#1 is the most likely, #2 is the second most likely, etc.). These triggers will be used to develop a plan for managing the unwanted behavior.

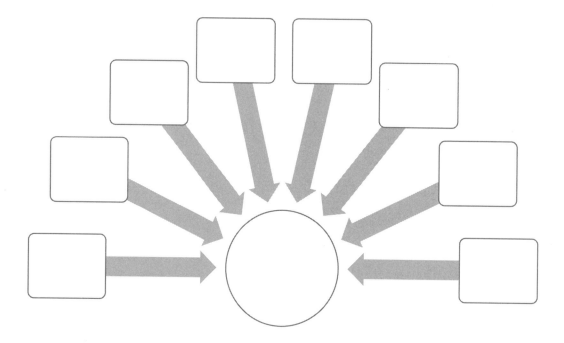

Treatment Plan

Complete this form with your practitioner. List any unwanted behavior or other concerns to be addressed in treatment in the first column. List your goals and objectives for each treatment target in the second column. Finally, list the treatment plan for each target in the third column. Many people find it helpful to address the top four triggers for each unwanted behavior in their plan. Revisions may be made throughout treatment as needed.

Target Behavior/ Symptom/Concern	Goals and Objectives	Treatment Plan

Three reasons why this plan is important to me:

1. _____

2. _____

3. _____

Change Plan for Assessment

My Plan to Get Started

Changes I would like to make:

_____

_____

_____

_____

These changes are important to me because:

_____

_____

_____

_____

_____

I plan to take these steps to get started (what, where, when, how):

_____

_____

_____

_____

_____

_____

IF this gets in the way   **THEN try this**

_____   _____

_____   _____

_____   _____

_____   _____

_____   _____

CHAPTER 4

Self-Monitoring

Self-monitoring, the process of clients observing and recording their own behaviors, thoughts, physiological sensations, or feelings, is a core component of CBT. Use self-monitoring as an assessment tool (as noted in the previous chapter) or as an intervention strategy in and of itself. Traditionally, self-monitoring of thoughts is an intervention strategy used early in CBT. A thought record tracks responses to situations and the links between thoughts, emotions, and behaviors (Beck, 2011, p. 195; Leahy, 2003, p. 8). Self-monitoring of antecedents and consequences of unwanted behaviors is also common in CBT (also known as "functional assessment" or "functional analysis"). Foundational to the treatment of anxiety disorders is the self-monitoring of distress, physiological symptoms, behavioral avoidance, and their triggers (Newman & Borkovec, 1995). The monitoring of activities, both pleasurable and distressful, is a cornerstone of behavioral activation for depression (Martell et al., 2010).

Across many fields of behavior change, there is consistent evidence that self-monitoring leads to improved outcome. For example, interventions that included self-monitoring resulted in improved adherence to HIV medication (Parsons et al., 2007; Safren et al., 2001). Meta-analyses have demonstrated that the self-monitoring of glucose levels and blood pressure lead to improved health outcomes (McIntosh et al., 2010; Uhlig, Patel, Ip, Kitsios, & Balk, 2013). Increased self-monitoring of food intake or physical activity is associated with positive response to weight loss interventions (Burke, Wang, & Sevick, 2011; Olander et al., 2013). Effective evidence-based interventions for substance use include self-monitoring to recognize cravings early and identify situational triggers (Fisher & Roget,

Self-monitoring leads to improved outcome.

2009, p. 930). When self-monitoring has been used as a baseline assessment, the effect on reducing drinking is significant enough that researchers have difficulty testing the effects of other interventions (Kavanagh, Sitharthan, Spilsbury, & Vignaendra, 1999; Sobell, Bogardis, Schuller, Leo, & Sobell, 1989). Other studies have found similar effects of self-monitoring on other behaviors (Humphreys, Marx, & Lexington, 2009). Despite its effectiveness, many clients are not fully adherent with self-monitoring (e.g., Newman, Consoli, & Taylor, 1999; Vincze, Barner, & Lopez, 2003). Integrating MI with CBT can help to improve adherence (Smith, Heckemeyer, Kratt, & Mason, 1997; Westra et al., 2009).

Engaging

Recall the three components that are a routine part of initial engagement for MI–CBT sessions: checking in on the client's previous change plan, setting the session agenda, and discussing the rationale for the session objectives. First, check in on the client's Change Plan from the previous week including any homework assignments. Refer to Chapter 7 for more details on managing difficulty with assignment completion. Using MI skills, affirm even small steps toward goal completion and any changes in the target concerns. Empathize with any goals not met and consider a minifunctional analysis for progress or lack thereof. Referring to the assessment chapter, you can briefly elicit the antecedents and consequences (or triggers and outcomes) of any successes or less-than-optimal goal completion and consider how to integrate this information into the ongoing treatment plan. In the following exchange, see how the practitioner quickly organizes Celia's description in terms of antecedents and consequences and implications for the treatment plan by using reflections and open questions.

> PRACTITIONER: You mentioned that you had a really bad day on Wednesday. [Reflect] Tell me a little more about that. [Open question]
>
> CELIA: I really had a hard time getting out of bed. The weather was rainy and I was scared to drive, so I called in sick to work. Then I felt really guilty that I was calling in again and that made me feel even worse.
>
> PRACTITIONER: So bad weather days bring up some fears. Calling in sick to work is the result, and then you feel so bad about that it makes the depression worse. [Reflect]
>
> CELIA: Yeah, then I can't get out of bed and I get even madder at myself.
>
> PRACTITIONER: It's a vicious cycle. So when we talk about managing triggers in the treatment plan, we can make sure we address how weather affects your activity and how guilty thoughts continue the cycle. [Action reflection to integrate treatment plan]

After discussing the previous week's goals, collaboratively set the session agenda with the client, exploring the rationale for agenda items to engage the client in the session. As described in the previous chapter, ask for permission, state planned session components, elicit feedback, reflect the feedback, and ask what the client would like to add. There are a few important points to keep track of here (see Table 4.1 for engaging guidelines). First, as a way of increasing engagement, tie the session agenda to the client's goals and change talk you have noticed in the previous session. Continue to use the word "*you*" to emphasize autonomy. Second, when engaging, the treatment tasks are discussed in general terms (e.g., "According to the treatment plan you made, today we were going to discuss how to keep track of things we are working on") rather than prescribing specifics of the task (e.g., "Today we are going to practice recording your mood every day for the next week"). In this way you leave room to collaboratively determine the specifics of self-monitoring during the focusing process. Third, when you sense that there may be ambivalence about the session agenda, it can be helpful to discuss the rationale immediately rather than waiting until after the agenda has been set, as demonstrated in the example below. When discussing the rationale for self-monitoring, you want to first elicit *what* the client knows about the task and then elicit *why* it might be important. Note that one part of the rationale of self-monitoring is that the data can be reviewed in subsequent sessions as information for assessment, treatment planning, or to monitor progress.

> First elicit *what* the client knows about the task, and then elicit *why* it might be important.

PRACTITIONER: You had said that a major concern is that you get anxious when you even consider speaking up in class, or when a professor may call on you. [Reflect]

SAM: Yes, I start to sweat, I can feel myself getting hot and I think my face gets red. I hate that. It is so embarrassing.

PRACTITIONER: OK, and you have one goal of reducing your anxiety in those situations. [Reflect to reinforce change talk]

SAM: Yes. I just wish that didn't happen.

PRACTITIONER: You want it to go away. [Reflect] OK, so we will work on this. One thing that can be helpful is monitoring this anxiety. What do you think that means? [Ask]

SAM: Like writing it down.

PRACTITIONER: Yes, like keeping track of it. One way is to write it down and later we can discuss some other ways so you can decide what's best for you. [Tell] Why might it be helpful to keep track? [Ask]

SAM: Well, I guess one reason would be to know if this treatment is working.

TABLE 4.1. Engaging Guidelines: Self-Monitoring

1. *Tie the session agenda to the client's goals and change talk noted in the previous session, emphasizing autonomy with "you" statements.*

   "You mentioned last time that your top priority is to stay healthy so that HIV doesn't interfere with your other life goals, like finishing school and supporting yourself with a job that allows you to use your creativity. So, our main focus for today will be on learning how to track your medication doses."

2. *Discuss treatment tasks in general terms rather than prescribing specifics of the task.*

   "Today, we will work on learning a skill that can help you to track your eating and activity patterns." (Specific terms are discussed during the focusing process.)

3. *Discuss rationales during agenda setting, rather than after, when ambivalence about the session agenda is detected* (first use ATA to elicit *what* the client knows; then *why* it might be important).

   THERAPIST: Today, we'll work on learning a skill to help you to keep track of patterns in your worries about safety. After that . . .

   CLIENT: (*interrupting*) Oh, I don't think that will work for me. It just happens and I don't even realize it until I'm already upset!

   THERAPIST: It's hard to picture yourself being able to keep track of worrying when you don't notice it starting. *What* do you already know about how people keep track of worries?

   CLIENT: Well, maybe they're more rational than I am when it's happening.

   THERAPIST: So, people who can recognize it happening earlier can be more successful at keeping track of their worries. (*pause*) I think you're onto something. When we talk about how to keep track, maybe we could think about some ways for you to notice the signs earlier too.

   CLIENT: I think I'll need that.

   THERAPIST: And *why* do you think it might be important to keep track of times when you worry?

   CLIENT: Well . . . I guess that's how we'd know when it is happening and when it isn't.

   THERAPIST: Great insight! Knowing when it is happening and when it isn't can really help us to figure out what to do about it, and what is and isn't working for you. What do you think?

   CLIENT: Maybe I can finally get this under control.

4. *Adhere to the engaging process goals of listening and understanding, avoiding planning, problem solving, skills training, and other CBT strategies during engaging.*

   THERAPIST: Today, we'll spend some time figuring out what helps and doesn't help you to take your antiretroviral medications each day.

   CLIENT: OK. I've been thinking that the one thing that gets in my way is not having a schedule to follow. I guess I could start keeping one.

   THERAPIST: You're already thinking about what you could do going forward. Let's make sure that we get that on the top of our list. If it's OK with you, before we start working on the steps you plan to take, could we spend a few minutes figuring out what other things affect the way you take your medications? That way, we can think about a few ways to set you up for success as you put your ideas into action.

   CLIENT: Sure. That sounds like a good idea.

5. *Consider the client's needs when deciding whether to use formal terms or lay terms to describe the session task* (use client language, or gauge how formally the client speaks in sessions and select your language accordingly).

   "You mentioned that you used to keep a *mood log.* How do you think doing something like that could help now?"

   "You mentioned that you used a phone app to *keep track of your moods.* How do you think doing something like that could help now?"

PRACTITIONER: Exactly. One major reason for monitoring anxiety is that we want to be able to tell if the treatment is working by learning about how severe, over time, your anxiety gets in these situations. [Tell] Are there other reasons that you can think of? [Ask]

SAM: Not sure. I know we talked about looking at how I think in anxiety-provoking situations.

PRACTITIONER: Yes, we had talked about how a critical component of CBT is the cognitive component. [Reflect] So the next part is that as you monitor the situations that make you anxious, we will want to look at what thoughts you are having during that situation. After you figure that out, we can come up with the best plan to manage the thought. [Tell]

Fourth, note that in the engaging process it is important to hold off on problem solving or other CBT strategies because the goal of engaging is to listen and understand. Problem-solving barriers can be addressed when the client is ready for the planning process. Although the processes are not sequential, premature planning can interfere with engaging, focusing, and evoking motivation. There will be time for problem solving potential barriers when you have addressed why to monitor, focused on how and what to monitor, and elicited and reinforced motivation for the task. Finally, it is your choice whether to use the official term of the task as "self-monitoring" or to use lay terms; and consider the needs of the client. In the case of Mary, an adolescent with weight loss concerns, the practitioner did not feel the need to use the word "self-monitoring" and instead uses terms like "keeping track" and later uses the term "logging."

PRACTITIONER: Are you ready to discuss the plan for our session today or is there more we should talk about in terms of how your week went? [Ask permission]

MARY: No, I think we got it.

PRACTITIONER: One of the things that could help you reach your weight loss goal so that you can feel better is to begin to keep track of your food and activity. So today we can spend some time thinking about how you want to do that. [Tell] When I say "keep track" what does that mean to you? [Ask about the "what" before the "why"]

MARY: I don't know because I can't write everything down all the time because I'm in school and I really don't want people to know what I am doing.

PRACTITIONER: So you're worried that keeping track means you have to write everything down in the moment. [Reflect] You're right that keeping track could mean writing things down when they happen like in a log, but there are a lot of options about how you do it, when you do it, and what exactly you do. We can talk about those later. [Tell and foreshadow the focusing process] For now, why do you think it would be important to keep track at all? [Ask]

MARY: I am really not sure. I mean I know sometimes you can eat more than you think you do.

PRACTITIONER: Right. You have noticed that keeping track helps you pay attention to what you eat, and studies have shown that just keeping track can help with some weight loss. [Reflect] Also, keeping track can help you figure out when you tend to overeat, what foods are involved, and what situations might be more tempting. [Tell] What do you think of those reasons for keeping track? [Ask]

MARY: Those make sense as long as I can figure out how to remember to do it. I usually forget by the end of the day. And if I am upset about something or watching TV, I definitely don't pay attention to what I eat!

PRACTITIONER: You have some concerns about how you will manage to do this. We can talk about those when we figure out exactly how you want to keep track. [Reflect and foreshadow the focusing and planning processes] For now, I just want to make sure we are on the same page about what we are going to do today, and it seems like keeping track of food is where you want to start. We can talk about keeping track of activity later. [Action reflection]

MARY: Yeah, that's fine. We can start with keeping track of food.

Sustain Talk and Discord

In Chapter 2, we introduced the concepts of sustain talk (statements against change) and discord (trouble in the relationship). We emphasized that sustain talk is a normal part of ambivalence. In the context of self-monitoring, sustain talk would sound like desire, ability, reasons, and need to avoid monitoring tasks. Some common statements include concerns about the time it will take to complete the task, about the task difficulty, about remembering to remember, and about disclosure when others may find out about the target concern or about treatment. Sometimes clients are concerned that self-monitoring will make them think about issues they are not ready to face, particularly when they are emotionally upsetting. The client may hesitate to admit to the level of concern, particularly for symptoms that he or she perceives as embarrassing (e.g., binge eating) or that have legal ramifications (e.g., substance use). Symptoms may also be protective (e.g., anxiety to ward off danger, eating to ward off sadness) and recording these symptoms is perceived as the first step in giving them up.

These issues and associated sustain talk are a *normal* part of the treatment process. As noted in Chapter 2, reflections can go a long way in responding to sustain talk and can strengthen the alliance. Emphasizing autonomy can reduce sustain talk. In addition to using *"you"* statements as in the example above, emphasizing freedom of choice is very powerful: "It's really up to you how much you want to keep track of things. I can suggest what works for most people, but you know best what will work for you." Ensuring that the client feels like there are options also reduces sustain talk: "There are lots of options you can consider in terms of what to record, how often to record, and what tools you might use." Offering options is different than problem solving in that you are just mentioning alternatives: "You could record on paper, or on your phone, or with some new apps." This is different from suggesting an alternative such as "You don't think you can remember, so maybe you can program your phone to remind you." The latter statement might come later with permission when focusing or planning.

Another issue relates to the protective aspect of symptoms. Clients can have a hard time imagining what it would be like to live without their symptoms. For example, anxiety can feel protective as a way of warding off danger. Avoidance of feared situations allows clients to feel comfortable in the short term, but have problems later because they miss out on things that they want in life. To help people get going, reassurance about monitoring can come into play: "All we are doing for this first step is keeping track of the symptoms. This will just help you to decide if and where you may want to make changes in the future. Keeping track of this could give you information to decide what you want to do, if anything. What do you think of that approach?"

If you ignore sustain talk or inadvertently fall into a mode of convincing or premature problem solving, you may experience discord. As described in Chapter 2, strategies to address discord include apologizing, affirming, and shifting focus. These can be combined—for example, you can apologize for pushing the client into something he or she is not ready to do, and then affirm the changes the client is willing to make: "You still want to stick with your goals, but recording your drinking is not something you are ready to do yet." Shifting focus is simply steering the conversation to a less controversial topic. You may need to drop self-monitoring for now and move on to other components of the treatment plan. (See "MI–CBT Dilemmas" below for more about this topic.)

Note that, for some behaviors, excessive self-monitoring can be detrimental. For example, in clients with obsessive–compulsive disorder (OCD), you would need to consider whether they are compulsively self-monitoring (Craske & Tsao, 1999). In clients with excessive worry, monitoring can be a way to maintain worry as a form of reassurance. Wilson and Vitousek (1999) caution against calorie counting for persons with anorexia or bulimia.

Focusing

In the focusing process you clarify what and how to monitor. We suggest reviewing the literature for your client's specific target concern in terms of how self-monitoring has been done within particular evidence-based treatments so that you have information you can provide within the context of ATA. There are many possible self-monitoring tools (see Client Handouts 4.1–4.5) that include questions to elicit change talk. Having some familiarity with new technology can also be helpful, as new options are emerging all the time. However, we have found that there is very little data on what self-monitoring options are associated with the best outcomes, so we say the best option is what the client is willing to do!

The first question is what to monitor. While this should be relatively clear based on the target concern, you and the client may need to determine how much information should be monitored at one time. For example, the client may monitor drinking episodes, amount of drinking, type of alcohol consumed, venue, or people involved. It is best to begin simply, collaboratively discussing the benefits and challenges of increasing the complexity of recording to develop the best plan. If goals are set too high, the client may abandon the goal in the face of failure (Marlatt & Gordon, 1985).

In terms of how to monitor, there are options regarding tools (written logs vs. technology-based approaches; forms vs. a notebook computer), as well as how often to monitor. For example, for behavioral activation for depression, Martell et al. (2010, pp. 70–71) described alternatives such as hour-by-hour monitoring, monitoring blocks of time during the day (recording takes place periodically recalling the previous 3–4 hours), and time sampling procedures (spot checks of behavior, as in Monday 1:00–3:00 P.M., Wednesday 8:00–11:00 A.M., and Saturday 6:00–9:00 P.M.). When behaviors take place less frequently, for example, with a client who binge drinks once or twice a week, the client may monitor drinking daily or may consider monitoring more frequent behaviors such as alcohol cravings or monitor drinking once a day at the end of the day.

As a general rule, first elicit ideas from the client before providing information. Ideas that come directly from the client may be more likely to be followed than those that you suggest. Of course, if you have concerns that clients are being unrealistic in terms of what they can manage, it is OK to express those concerns with permission. The exploration of these options and focusing in on a particular self-monitoring approach is all done with ATA and reflections as in the case of Eugene below.

> PRACTITIONER: We talked about what monitoring is and you said it was important to help you keep track of how you are doing with your medications. Now if it's OK with you, we can decide specifically what you want to monitor and how you want to do this. [Ask]

EUGENE: I have to take my medications twice a day, once in the morning and once at night.

PRACTITIONER: So you need to keep track of morning and evening doses. [Reflect] How would you like to do that? [Ask] Some people prefer in the moment, and some prefer at the end of the day. [Tell]

EUGENE: In the moment might be better for remembering, but I don't really want to mess with my day.

PRACTITIONER: So you would like to do it at the end of the day as long as you have a way of remembering. [Reflect] What ideas do you have about a monitoring system that would work for you? [Ask]

EUGENE: I think using my phone would be the best bet. I could program an alarm or something and then record it in my notes.

PRACTITIONER: You have some solid ideas about using your phone. [Reflect] There might be some new apps around for keeping track of medications also. [Tell]

EUGENE: I could check out some of those.

PRACTITIONER: So what do you think about starting with your idea for now— setting an alarm at the end of the day and then recording in your notes whether you took your meds in the morning and at night? [Ask] We could add exploring other apps to your weekly plan later if you want. [Emphasize autonomy]

EUGENE: Sounds like a plan, but I better program the phone right now or I won't remember later.

PRACTITIONER: You're good at doing things right away to help you remember. [Affirming reflection] There are other things people track like who they were with or how they were feeling, like triggers, especially if they missed. What do you think about tracking that stuff? [Ask]

EUGENE: I don't know if I'm ready for that.

PRACTITIONER: So you would prefer to start with the simple yes or no for A.M. and P.M. [Reflect] and then if we need to later we can consider adding the other information. [Action reflection]

Evoking

Once you have focused on what and how to self-monitor, open questions should elicit change talk for that specific target (e.g., "Why is it important to you to use your phone app to track your drinking every day?"; "What's the best thing that can happen if you are able to get a complete week of logging your food at the end of each day?"). Motivation is at the intersection of importance and confidence (Miller & Rollnick, 2012), and as you move into more structured CBT tasks, evoking confidence becomes increasingly important. CBT has emphasized the importance of efficacy beliefs, the confidence and optimism about the effectiveness of the interventions and about one's ability to follow treatment recommendations (Lynch, Vansteenkiste, Deci, & Ryan, 2011). MI has specified several strategies to support self-efficacy. Affirming reflections, reflections of positive qualities or strengths in the person, is one such strategy ("You have been very persistent in trying to get off probation"). You can tie these affirmations to the current target behavior ("And this persistence might help you stick to your recording goal").

Exploring Personal Strengths

There are several types of questions that support the client's self-efficacy. One type uses encouraging stories regarding past successes directly related to the task at hand: "You mentioned you used to keep track of how much you spent every day when you were short on cash. How did you remember to do that?" You may also explore other challenges and use the strengths elicited in an affirming reflection ("You mentioned you managed to keep the job at the gas station even though nobody helped you with transportation. How did you overcome this challenge?"). Similarly, you can inquire about successfully accomplished goals from the past, personal strengths, or social supports available to help with overcoming challenges (e.g., "Who helped you? What are the things you did that made a difference?").

For the client who does not easily identify personal strengths, consider exploring what other people (e.g., friends, family) say about the person's strengths or good qualities. Try a structured activity where the client chooses from an array of strengths listed on a worksheet as shown in Client Handout 4.6 or on a stack of cards (e.g., thoughtful, kind, strong). Then follow up with open questions about how these qualities are currently evident in the client's life, both in relation to past successes and to the task at hand—for example: "You mentioned you've always been a strong person. How might being a strong person help you if you decided to . . . ?"

Using a Ruler

Previous chapters have described the use of a scale to increase commitment, and similarly the use of a ruler is often incorporated into MI interventions (Miller & Rollnick, 2012). After asking permission, describe or show a picture of the "ruler," with anchors of 1 as the lowest and 10 as the highest, as shown in Client Handout 4.7. Then ask the client to rate on the ruler's scale, from 1 to 10, "How confident are you that you can . . . ?" After the client chooses a number, the first task is to reflect the response. Second, ask why he or she did not pick a *lower* number. By inquiring about lower numbers, you increase the likelihood of the person responding with change talk about ability. That is, you are guiding the person to defend a position with statements of self-efficacy instead of stating why he or she is not confident. Note that if the person responds that he or she is a 1 on the ruler, this is a clue to you about reconsidering the plan. These steps are demonstrated in the following example.

PRACTITIONER: If it's OK with you I'd like to find out how confident you're feeling about using this logging form to keeping track of your cravings and your drinking next week.

CARL: OK

PRACTITIONER: So, on a 10-point scale, some people feel not at all confident when starting this process and rate a 1. A few people rate a 10 because they have done it before and are completely confident. Others might be in the middle like a 4, 5, or 6. Where are you at?

CARL: Probably a 5.

PRACTITIONER: You are somewhere in the middle. You have some confidence you can do this but you are not sure. Why did you say a 5 and not a lower number?

CARL: Well, I really want to get off probation and I know I am going to screw up if I don't get a handle on this. So, if I set my mind to it, I think I can do it.

PRACTITIONER: OK, so when you set your mind to something, you feel you can make it happen. [Affirming reflection] In this treatment, writing down the triggers and cravings will help you get a handle on things, and should help you get off probation. [Action reflection]

TIP for Rulers: Ask What It Would Take to Get to a Higher Number

The question "What would it take to get to a higher number?" helps to identify sources of increased self-efficacy and begins to move to the planning process as the client thinks about what else needs to happen to complete the task.

PRACTITIONER: You said you were about a 5 for how confident you are to log your drinking, cravings, and triggers. What would it take for you to choose a higher number?

CARL: I guess if I could make up some reminder system, I might be higher. I am worried I will forget, especially when things get crazy at home.

Planning

While the focusing process addressed how and what to monitor with some specificity, in the planning process the client will specify the steps for implementation. Recall the Change Plan from the previous chapters that included restating the goal, specifying the steps to reach that goal, identifying barriers, and delineating plans to overcome these barriers. Specifying the steps moves the conversation beyond the details of the logging process and addresses how to integrate self-monitoring into the client's daily life (see Client Handout 4.8 and Figure 4.1 for a sample Change Plan). The research literature calls this process the "formation of implementation

---

My Plan for Keeping Track

Changes I would like to make:

Start taking my medication every day

Don't miss any clinic appointments

Manage my health so that I can stay healthy

These changes are important to me because:

I do not want to die young

I do not want to become sick and unable to take care of myself

I want my parents to see that I am taking care of myself

I do not want to infect someone

How keeping track can help me:

If I write it down, I can remember better. I can see when I usually miss my
medications.

I plan to take these steps to keep track (what, where, when, how):

Make taking my medication part of my daily routine by putting it on my schedule

Recording when I take my medication every day before I go to bed.

IF this gets in the way	THEN try this
I forget to make a list of triggers	Put a reminder in my phone calendar
I do not have my medication with me when it is time to take it	Take it as soon as possible; carry 1 day's dose with me whenever I can
I don't have any privacy to complete my log sheet	Send myself a message on my phone and record it later
I do not feel like taking my medication	Remind myself of why it is important and how it will help me to stay healthy

---

FIGURE 4.1. Eugene's Change Plan for self-monitoring.

intentions" (Gollwitzer, 1999), the identification of specific triggers to perform a specific action. We refer to them as "when–then" plans ("*When* I brush my teeth, *then* I will record my mood"). Thus, first you guide the client to form a when–then plan or implementation intention, then you review the barriers and form an if–then plan ("If I lose my log, then I will e-mail myself the information and transfer it later"). You can also ask the client to describe a typical weekday and weekend day to help to determine how to implement self-monitoring in a real-world context.

PRACTITIONER: Last time you described a typical day from the beginning to the end, and I am wondering how you think this recording plan will fit into your day. [Open question]

CELIA: The morning is pretty hectic getting everyone off to school, so I am going to have to do it before I even get going. I usually have lots of bad thoughts when I first wake up anyway.

PRACTITIONER: So when you wake up in the morning, then you can see yourself completing the thought record before you get downstairs and make everyone breakfast. [Reflection and when–then plan] How will you continue the log during the day? [Open question]

CELIA: Probably when I get to work.

PRACTITIONER: OK, so you will continue the record at work. [Reflect] What might get in the way? [Open question to elicit barriers]

CELIA: I might forget it and I might not want anyone at work to see what I am doing.

PRACTITIONER: Forgetting to keep the paper with you and worrying about others seeing what you are doing could get in the way. [Reflect] How can you get over this barrier? [Open question]

CELIA: I am not sure.

PRACTITIONER: If it's OK with you we can discuss some options. [Ask for permission to offer information with menu of options]

CELIA: If you have any ideas, let me know.

PRACTITIONER: Some people keep the log somewhere where they will always have it, like in a purse or folded in their phone case since you said you would rather a paper-and-pencil version. [Tell] What do you think about those options for keeping it with you? [Ask]

CELIA: I think the purse will work, but I don't know how to keep everyone out of my business. But you know, I usually take my purse to the bathroom so I could fill it out there.

PRACTITIONER: You have some ideas about how to make this work. [Affirming reflection] Keeping the log in your purse would keep it with you at all times and if you don't have privacy, then you can go to the bathroom with your purse to complete it. [If–then plan).

Be cautious if the client is not able to identify barriers. Polivy and Herman (2002) discuss an important point about self-efficacy. They define the "false hope syndrome" as "unrealistic expectations about the likely speed, amount, ease, and consequences of self-change attempts" (p. 677). Overconfidence and setting unrealistic goals often undermines successful change. You may guide the client toward a more realistic plan by suggesting barriers with permission in a menu of options ("Some clients have said that they struggle with remembering to log, with other people seeing them log, or forgetting details about what happened. How might those things apply to you?"). Even if the client denies these barriers now, he or she

> First you guide the client to form a *when–then* plan, then you review the barriers and form an *if–then* plan.

will recall the discussion if he or she struggles during the week and be more ready for a plan the following week. If the client agrees, elicit his or her ideas to overcoming barriers before providing the client with a menu of options.

> **TIP for Planning: Use Visualization to Enhance Goal Attainment**
>
> The research literature suggests that visualizing the link between a situation and a goal (When this happens, I will do this) is more likely to result in goal completion than verbal commitment only (Gollwitzer & Sheeran, 2006). Others have noted that prospective memory (remembering to remember to complete an action in the future) is improved when individuals imagine themselves performing the action in response to a future cue (Chasteen, Park, & Schwarz, 2001). Thus, guiding clients to visualize components of their Change Plan may improve the likelihood of completion beyond verbal formation of the plan. Visualization can be done by simply asking the client, with permission, to imagine and describe the situation and his or her intended behavior. Alternatively, visualization can be done more formally with guided imagery where
>
> > Guiding the client to visualize components of his or her Change Plan may improve the likelihood of completion.
>
> you guide the client to use all senses to imagine the cue–behavior link in a relaxed state, as in Client Handout 4.9 (Andersson & Moss, 2011; Utay & Miller, 2006).

MI–CBT Dilemmas

The key dilemma is how to manage when the client is not ready to engage in self-monitoring and you believe it is a critical ingredient for successful treatment. There are some choices. You may inform the client that self-monitoring is necessary for the CBT you provide and that if the client is not ready to complete the task, then he or she may not be ready for CBT. As described in the previous chapter, you may decide to see the client for MI-only sessions or have him or her return to see you when he or she is ready to engage in CBT with self-monitoring. Alternatively, you can decide to provide MI–CBT without self-monitoring, perhaps asking the client to revisit the idea if progress is not sufficient. Finally, you may try to negotiate alternatives to full monitoring such as brief yes-or-no checklists, a call or text check-in during the week to elicit target information, or a recall interview at the beginning of the next session.

ACTIVITY 4.1 FOR PRACTITIONERS

The Experience of Self-Monitoring

Self-monitoring in some form appears to be an important ingredient for successful CBT, but it isn't easy! Common complaints include lack of time, forgetting, lack of privacy, and simply not wanting to deal with target concerns on a regular basis as required for monitoring. MI skills can help to build the client's intrinsic motivation for self-monitoring assignments.

ACTIVITY GOAL: In this activity you observe your own self-monitoring so that you can experience and understand how your clients might feel. You can experience the links between motivation (importance and confidence) and completion of monitoring assignments.

ACTIVITY INSTRUCTIONS: Choose two behaviors you are thinking about changing, one behavior that you are more ready to change and one that you are less ready to change. Now rate each behavior on the following scales:

Behavior 1: _____

Importance Ruler: Mark on the ruler how important you feel this behavior is to change.

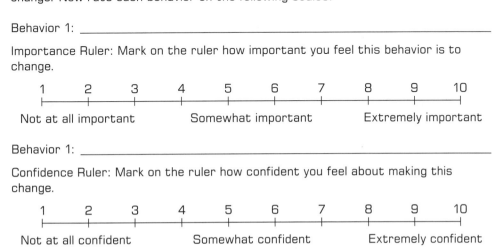

Behavior 1: _____

Confidence Ruler: Mark on the ruler how confident you feel about making this change.

Behavior 2: _____

Importance Ruler: Mark on the ruler how important you feel this behavior is to change.

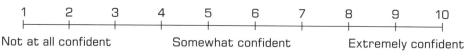

Not at all important   Somewhat important   Extremely important

Behavior 2: _____

Confidence Ruler: Mark on the ruler how confident you feel about making this change.

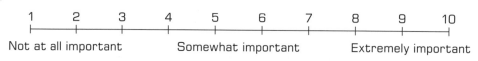

Not at all confident   Somewhat confident   Extremely confident

Now make a plan to monitor each behavior. You can choose which behavior to monitor first or decide to monitor both at the same time. Decide exactly what and how you are going to do this. If possible, try to monitor each behavior for at least a few days. If completing this activity in a group or with a partner, you may have your partner guide you in a 3-day recall of each behavior instead.

My Plan for Behavior 1

Importance Ruler: Mark on the ruler how important you feel this self-monitoring plan for Behavior 1 is to do.

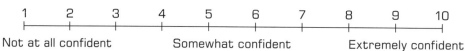

Not at all important   Somewhat important   Extremely important

Confidence Ruler: Mark on the ruler how confident you feel about completing this plan for Behavior 1.

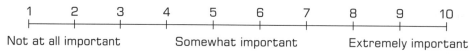

Not at all confident   Somewhat confident   Extremely confident

My Plan for Behavior 2

Importance Ruler: Mark on the ruler how important you feel this self-monitoring plan for Behavior 2 is to do.

Not at all important   Somewhat important   Extremely important

Confidence Ruler: Mark on the ruler how confident you feel about completing this plan for Behavior 2.

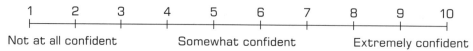

Not at all confident   Somewhat confident   Extremely confident

After 3 or more days of self-monitoring, consider the following questions.

For Behavior 1, how hard or easy was it to complete monitoring for each behavior?

_____

_____

_____

For Behavior 1, what were the barriers and facilitators to completing the task for each behavior?

_____

_____

_____

For Behavior 2, how hard or easy was it to complete monitoring for each behavior?

_____

_____

_____

For Behavior 2, what were the barriers and facilitators to completing the task for each behavior?

_____

_____

_____

What did you notice about the relationships between the first set of rulers (importance and confidence for behavior change) and the second set of rulers (importance and confidence for self-monitoring)?

_____

_____

_____

What did you notice about your ratings on the rulers for behavior change (first set of rulers) and how you completed the tasks?

_____

_____

_____

What did you notice about your ratings on the rulers for self-monitoring and how you completed the tasks?

_____

_____

_____

Sequences: Eliciting and Reinforcing Change Talk for Self-Monitoring

ACTIVITY GOAL: In this activity you will practice developing evoking questions to elicit change talk specifically for self-monitoring. You will then develop a reflection to reinforce the change talk.

ACTIVITY INSTRUCTIONS: For each of the following items, fill in the blanks, making up additional details of the case as necessary. You will practice completing each of the three components of the sequences. In the first section, you will complete one of the three components of the sequence (question to elicit change talk, client change talk, reflection of change talk). In the second section, you will use your creativity to complete two of the three components.

Item 1

- **Practitioner Strategy to Elicit Change Talk:** What can you do to keep track of your calories?
- **Client Change Talk:** I could write down what I eat and drink every day. My aunt does that to keep track of her calories, and she lost a lot of weight.

- **Practitioner Reinforcement (Reflection/Question):** _____

_____

Item 2

- **Practitioner Strategy to Elicit Change Talk:** Why would it be important to you to keep a daily food log?

- **Client Change Talk:** _____

_____

- **Practitioner Reinforcement (Reflection/Question):** It's important to you because, if you have the right information, you can make healthy choices.

Item 3

- **Practitioner Strategy to Elicit Change Talk:** _____

_____

- **Client Change Talk:** I'll start tomorrow morning.
- **Practitioner Reinforcement (Reflection/Question):** Right away.

Item 4

- **Practitioner Strategy to Elicit Change Talk:** Eugene, now that we've talked about using a log to keep track of whether you've taken your daily medications, what's the best thing that could happen if you log every day?

- **Client Change Talk:** _____

_____

- **Practitioner Reinforcement (Reflection/Question):** _____

_____

Item 5

- **Practitioner Strategy to Elicit Change Talk:** _____

- **Client Change Talk:** I've been able to manage my work schedule and my class schedule. So, I do know how to stay organized—even though I missed my clinic appointment.
- **Practitioner Reinforcement (Reflection/Question):** _____

_____

Item 6

- **Practitioner Strategy to Elicit Change Talk:** _____

_____

- **Client Change Talk:** _____

_____

- **Practitioner Reinforcement (Reflection/Question):** Making it part of your routine is the key.

Suggested Responses

Item 1
- **Practitioner Reinforcement (Reflection/Question):** You can picture yourself keeping a food log for weight loss too.

Item 2
- **Client Change Talk:** Because writing down what I eat and drink each day will help me to know where my calories are coming from and what my food weaknesses are. Maybe it will help my mom to see that I have trouble with certain foods too.

Item 3
- **Practitioner Strategy to Elicit Change Talk:** When would you want to start keeping a log?

Item 4
- **Client Change Talk:** I could be a healthier person. Also, I'd have a better idea of when I'm about to run out of medication.
- **Practitioner Reinforcement (Reflection/Question):** You'd not only feel healthier, but you'd be able to plan ahead so that you can stay healthy.

Item 5

- **Practitioner Strategy to Elicit Change Talk:** What personal strengths do you have that can help you to remember to fill out your log every day?
- **Practitioner Reinforcement (Reflection/Question):** You know what it takes to plan ahead and manage your responsibilities.

Item 6

- **Practitioner Strategy to Elicit Change Talk:** How do you see yourself using that strength to help with your medication management?
- **Client Change Talk:** I need to make it part of my routine. I could just put it on my schedule and then I wouldn't forget.

Self-Monitoring Wallet Card

Keeping track of unwanted behavior can help you with preventing it or managing it. It can also help you to evaluate your progress over time. This wallet card can be carried with you to assist you with keeping track of unwanted behavior. Cut out the card below and keep it in your wallet or purse.

	MINI MINDER		
	PLACE ONE MARK IN THE SPACE EACH TIME		
	_____ OCCURS		
M		F	
TU		SA	
W		SU	
TH		WHAT CHOICES WILL YOU MAKE TODAY TO REACH YOUR GOAL?	

How Did I Manage?

Keeping track of how you respond to unwanted behavior can help you with preventing it or managing it. This log can also help you to evaluate your progress over time. Complete this log each time _____ occurs.

Date/Time	Emotion	What I Did to Manage the Emotion	Was This Helpful? Why or Why Not?
Example: Monday/ 4:00 P.M.	*Example:* Anger	*Example:* I was angry with my brother. I went for a walk to get away.	*Example:* Yes. I didn't feel as angry when I got home, and the walk helped me think of other ideas.

Self-Monitoring Food Log

Keeping track of what you eat and drink can help you with making healthy changes as you identify patterns related to types of food and beverages, times of the day, and so on. This log can also help you to evaluate your progress over time. Complete this log every day (including the questions at the bottom), totaling your calories for the day at the bottom.

Date: _____   My Daily Calorie Goal: _____

When did I eat today?	What did I eat and drink today?	How much did I eat?	Where did the food come from *and* how was it prepared?	How many calories?
(Time of day that you ate)	(bread, rolls, buns, crackers, cookies, cheese, chips, milk, butter, jam, dressing, veggies, fruit, toppings, dessert, drinks, regular, light, low fat, low calorie/sugar)	(cup, tbsp, tsp, size of a fist, ½ baseball, deck of cards, whole bag, can/bottle)	(my house, grandma's house, restaurant [name], school, convenience store; baked, fried, grilled, boiled, raw, no skin)	(use the food label, review your calorie counter book, look online)
			Total Calories:	

What were my strengths today? _____

_____

What am I going to do differently based on this log? _____

_____

Three reasons why keeping a food log is important to me:

1. _____

2. _____

3. _____

Self-Monitoring Activity Log

Keeping track of your daily activity and screen time can help you with making healthy changes as you identify patterns related to types of activity, times of the day, how vigorous the activity is, and the like. This log can also help you to evaluate your progress over time. Complete this log every day, entering calories burned and screen time for the week at the bottom.

Date: _____   My Daily Activity Goal: _____

	What lifestyle activities and exercise did I do today?	How long did I do the activity or exercise?	How vigorous was the activity or exercise?	Total Calories Burned for Week / Calories burned for activity or exercise	How much screen time did I have?
	(List the activity/exercise you did for each day)	(Write down how long you did the activity/exercise—5 min? 30 min?)	(Circle the level of intensity for each activity/exercise—easy (E), moderate (M), vigorous (V))	(Write the calories burned for each activity/exercise)	(Circle one TV for each 30 minutes of screen time—including TV, computer, tablet, and phone screen time)
Monday			E M V		🖥 🖥 🖥 🖥
			E M V		🖥 🖥 🖥 🖥
			E M V		🖥 🖥 🖥 🖥
Tuesday			E M V		🖥 🖥 🖥 🖥
			E M V		🖥 🖥 🖥 🖥
			E M V		🖥 🖥 🖥 🖥
Wednesday			E M V		🖥 🖥 🖥 🖥
			E M V		🖥 🖥 🖥 🖥
			E M V		🖥 🖥 🖥 🖥
Thursday			E M V		🖥 🖥 🖥 🖥
			E M V		🖥 🖥 🖥 🖥
			E M V		🖥 🖥 🖥 🖥
Friday			E M V		🖥 🖥 🖥 🖥
			E M V		🖥 🖥 🖥 🖥
			E M V		🖥 🖥 🖥 🖥

(continued)

Self-Monitoring Activity Log (page 2 of 2)

	What lifestyle activities and exercise did I do today?	How long did I do the activity or exercise?	How vigorous was the activity or exercise?	Total Calories Burned for Week / Calories burned for activity or exercise	How much screen time did I have?
Saturday			E M V E M V E M V		
Sunday			E M V E M V E M V		
			Totals		

What are my strengths this week? _____

_____

_____

_____

_____

_____

_____

_____

_____

What am I going to do differently based on this log? _____

_____

_____

_____

_____

_____

_____

_____

_____

_____

Self-Monitoring Caregiver Support

Reviewing your child's daily food and activity logs can help you to stay informed about his or her progress and to identify times when your guidance is especially needed. This log can also help you to evaluate your child's progress over time. Complete this log at least once a week, while reviewing your child's food and activity logs. It can be helpful to review this form with your child, highlighting his or her strengths and offering guidance in the one or two areas where it is most needed.

What are the three most important reasons for me to look at my child's food and activity logs at least once a week?

1. _____

2. _____

3. _____

How do I see myself being helpful to my child? _____

_____

Food Log	Mon	Tues	Wed	Thur	Fri	Sat	Sun
Date that food was eaten was recorded							
Times that food was eaten was recorded							
Foods eaten were described well (portion size, type, prep method)							
Calories were written for each food							

Activity Log	Mon	Tues	Wed	Thur	Fri	Sat	Sun
Date of activity/exercise was recorded							
Times of activity/exercise was recorded							
Activity/exercise was described well (length of time, easy/moderate/vigorous)							
Calories burned were written for each activity/exercise							

What strengths or improvements did I notice on my child's logs? _____

_____

What did I see that told me that my child needs extra help or support? _____

_____

What am I going to do this week to help my child be successful? _____

_____

Personal Strengths

Check off each of your strengths, including the ones that you think only apply sometimes or in certain situations.

☐ Spontaneous	☐ Tolerant
☐ Compassionate	☐ Wise
☐ Emotional	☐ Warm
☐ Enthusiastic	☐ Optimistic
☐ Persistent	☐ Organized
☐ Honest	☐ Thoughtful
☐ Ethical	☐ Logical
☐ Intuitive	☐ Passionate
☐ Concise	☐ Curious
☐ Precise	☐ Flexible
☐ Discrete	☐ Generous
☐ Careful	☐ Peaceful
☐ Tender	☐ Intelligent
☐ Realistic	☐ Calm
☐ Imaginative	☐ Understanding
☐ Patient	☐ Exuberant
☐ Daring	☐ Fun
☐ Thorough	☐ Trustworthy
☐ Spirited	☐ Moderate
☐ Encouraging	☐ Creative
☐ Secure	

Commitment Ruler

On a scale from 1 to 10, where 1 is "not at all committed" and 10 is "extremely committed," how committed are you to _____
to help you make the changes you want to make?

1	2	3	4	5	6	7	8	9	10

Not at all committed   Somewhat committed   Extremely committed

You chose a _____. List three reasons why you chose this number and not a *lower* number.

1. _____

   _____

   _____

2. _____

   _____

   _____

3. _____

   _____

   _____

What would it take for you to get to a *higher* number (or to stay at a 10 if you are already there)? _____

_____

_____

_____

_____

_____

_____

_____

_____

_____

Change Plan for Self-Monitoring

My Plan for Keeping Track

Changes I would like to make:

_____

_____

_____

_____

These changes are important to me because:

_____

_____

_____

_____

How keeping track can help me:

_____

_____

_____

_____

I plan to take these steps to keep track (what, where, when, how):

_____

_____

_____

_____

IF this gets in the way	THEN try this
_____	_____
_____	_____
_____	_____
_____	_____
_____	_____

Visual Script for Encoding a Plan

People use their imagination to picture themselves walking through each step of a task that they want to do better at or want to remember better. For example, you might have heard about athletes like baseball players using this method to improve their swing. Another example is visualizing all the things you want to remember to buy at the store before you leave the house. So, by actually *picturing* each step of what needs to happen, you're more likely to get this into your brain to remember *what needs to happen when*.

How do you think that this kind of visualizing might be helpful with your recording plan?

_____

_____

_____

_____

So we are going to practice this. Walk through the actual steps of the plan you just created. While doing this, visualize the steps, as if you actually need to get to your sessions right now. We want this to be as vivid in your mind as possible, so I will be asking you to picture what you would see, hear, or feel during this time.

Remember, your plan was to _____

_____

(e.g., "When I brush my teeth at night, I will finish my recording log").

1. Close your eyes since we will be imagining the actual process and steps.
2. Take a deep breath to focus your attention and calm yourself. Now take another deep breath.
3. Now relax your body. Pay attention to you breathing as you relax your body.
4. Imagine that you are have going to brush your teeth before bed.
   - What time would it usually be and where would you be?
   - What would you usually be doing?
   - Try to picture the area where you would be as clearly as possible.
   - What do you smell?
   - Do you hear anything?
   - What do you hear?
   - The more you use your other senses (touch, smell, and hearing), the clearer the image will be for you.

(continued)

5. Now, imagine you are thinking about your log when you brush. What do you need to do now? Practice saying the reasons why you want to record sessions to make some changes in your life. Now imagine that as you finish brushing your teeth you are going to complete your log. Imagine the steps you will take to get to do this (e.g., find your phone, open the notes page, complete the log). Let's go through each step to make sure you do not miss any. Think of all the sounds, smells, and senses (e.g., feel of the phone, typing on the screen).

6. OK, take a deep breath and open your eyes. Great job of practicing visualizing your plan!

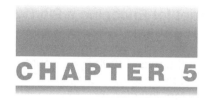

CHAPTER 5

Cognitive Skills

CBT is an educative treatment through which clients learn cognitive, behavioral, and emotional regulation skills. Over time clients can transition to being their own counselor and, ideally, these learned skills become automatic (see *www.beck-institute.org*). This chapter addresses cognitive skills through which clients learn to think more adaptively. The next chapter addresses behavioral and emotional regulation skills. Skills training may be the area where integrating MI and CBT integration is most important. A key component of CBT is to help clients learn how to evaluate and change long-standing behaviors. A key component of MI is to help clients resolve ambivalence about changing difficult behaviors. Generally speaking, in MI–CBT integration, cognitive, behavioral, and emotional regulation skills can be addressed in any order based on the collaboratively developed treatment plan. We present cognitive skills first only because it is central to the cognitive model, and because cognitive restructuring is often necessary before a client is ready to try new behavioral and emotion regulation skills. More behavioral approaches (Anton et al., 2006; Dimidjian et al., 2006; Naar-King et al., 2016) emphasize starting with behavioral and emotional regulation skills, and addressing cognitive skills as an adjunct as necessary.

Recall that orientation to CBT emphasizes the degree to which negative thoughts and beliefs govern the interpretation of situations. These interpretations in turn result in how one behaves and how one responds emotionally, creating or maintaining a cycle of distress. Changing thoughts leads to changes in beliefs and in how situations are interpreted. Accordingly, the management of thoughts is central to changing distressing emotions, as well as the behaviors that maintain these emotions (Beck, 2011). To help a client to manage thoughts adaptively, treatment focuses on "cognitive restructuring," a term referring to the range of strategies that help the client recognize, challenge, and modify unhelpful thoughts and beliefs. The components of cognitive restructuring include (1) education regarding the links between situations, thoughts, behaviors, and emotions (engaging the client in the intervention); (2) identification and categorization of negative thoughts (focusing on the thoughts most relevant for the client); (3) exploration and challenging of those negative thoughts through Socratic dialogue and hypothesis testing (a process of questioning and probing to stimulate critical thinking); and (4) developing between-session plans to continue the restructuring process in the real world (planning for restructuring). Thus, we refer to Step 1 in the engagement process, Step 2 in the focusing process, Step 3 in the evoking process, and Step 4 in the planning process. (See Table 5.1.) Recall, however, that the four processes and the associated components of cognitive restructuring do not need to occur sequentially within the session and may not all happen within a single session. The client and you may weave in and out of these steps as you explore different situations and patterns as well as events from the preceding week.

Engaging

After checking in on the client's change plan from the previous week, including homework and reviewing any outcome measures for progress, you collaboratively set the session agenda as described in previous chapters by asking for permission, stating potential session components, eliciting feedback, reflecting that feedback, and asking what the client would like to modify or add to the agenda. Cognitive restructuring may have been prioritized as part of the initial treatment plan, or you and the client may determine that cognitive restructuring strategies are needed because of events that occurred during the previous week. For example, Carl had a particularly bad week with drinking cravings related to feelings of hopelessness. As you listen with reflections and open questions, it becomes clear that cognitive restructuring strategies may need to take precedence over other skills training approaches originally prioritized in the treatment plan. You and Carl collaboratively decide the agenda.

> CARL: This week sucked. NFL season opener, and I'm not supposed to drink. I had three shots and then made myself throw up. I might as well turn myself in. I am never going to be able to finish probation.
>
> PRACTITIONER: You had a really rough week. Lots of temptation and it feels hopeless. [Reflect]
>
> CARL: Yeah, I just don't know if I can do this. I just want to run away and drink myself to sleep.

TABLE 5.1. Cognitive Restructuring: Four Steps

1. *Engaging:* Education regarding the links between situations, thoughts, behaviors, and emotions (engaging in the intervention).

   Sample applications:
   - Set the agenda.
   - Discuss rationales.
     - Use ATA to elicit *what* the client knows and *why* it might be important.
     - Lay the groundwork for the *focusing* process by addressing how thoughts create feelings and how thoughts differ from facts.
   - Return to the engaging process as needed when working on challenging thoughts and beliefs, or sustain talk and discord.

2. *Focusing:* Identification and categorization of negative thoughts (focusing on the thoughts most relevant for the client).

   Sample applications:
   - Ask permission to assist the client with identifying automatic thoughts and core beliefs.
     - Guide the client in use of visualization.
     - Role-play the situation.
     - Elicit the meaning of the situation from the client.
     - Offer a menu of options (helpful/unhelpful thoughts).
   - Avoid the expert trap by emphasizing autonomy.
     - Elicit client ideas and observations on potential thinking patterns.
     - Collaboratively name the patterns.

3. *Evoking:* Exploration and challenging of those thoughts through Socratic dialogue and hypothesis testing (a process of questioning and probing to stimulate critical thinking).

   Sample applications:
   - Use Socratic questioning collaboratively for the purpose of guided discovery.
     - Listen, summarize, and ask synthesizing or analytical questions.
       - Use open questions, reflective listening, summarizing, and asking a key question.
   - Evoke importance and confidence during cognitive restructuring work.
     - Use open questions, rulers, reflections, and affirmations of strengths.

4. *Planning:* Development of between-session plans to continue the restructuring process in the real world (planning for restructuring).

   Sample applications:
   - Move from whether and why to change thinking to *how* to change thinking.
     - Recall that this is not necessarily separated from the other processes.
   - Guide the client in:
     - Making a plan for change.
       - Evaluate between-session thoughts.
       - Develop alternative thoughts.
       - Develop self-statements.
     - Focusing on between-session activities.
       - Conduct behavioral experiments to test thoughts.
       - Practice graduated exposure—mutually agree on steps to take to face the avoided or feared situations.
       - Assist the client with planning for different outcomes of the plan for change.
     - Consolidating commitment to the plan.
       - Develop action steps including implementation intentions.
       - Identify potential barriers to implementation.
       - Generate solutions to potential barriers.
       - Elicit commitment language.
       - Assist in generating a rationale response/coping statement to be used during difficult situations.

PRACTITIONER: When you have hopeless thoughts it makes you want to quit trying. [Reflect] I am wondering if you would like to focus on the thoughts today instead of some of the skills practice that we planned. What do you think? [Open question]

CARL: I don't know. What do you think?

PRACTITIONER: It is really up to you, but if you are feeling hopeless you may not feel like practicing the skills. It might feel like "What's the point?," so it would make sense to talk about that. But if practicing skills makes you feel like there is hope, then we could continue with that plan. [Offer options]

CARL: Maybe the hopeless feelings first, then skills after.

Discussing the Rationale for Cognitive Restructuring

Recall that engagement while setting the session agenda includes discussing (not providing!) the rationale. In the last chapter we suggested a few communication tips to increase engagement: tie the session agenda to previous change talk, use the word "*you*" to emphasize autonomy, and discuss the treatment tasks in general terms, waiting to collaboratively determine specifics until the focusing process. It is also important to hold off on problem solving as the goal of engaging is to listen and understand. In our experience, jumping into skills training in CBT before the client is ready is one of the key mistakes of the novice CBT therapist, and potentially a key reason for clients not staying engaged in care or not completing exercises outside of sessions. It is particularly important when attempting to

> Hold off on problem solving; the goal of engaging is to listen and understand.

follow a treatment manual; you need to make sure that you are not on chapter 8, while the client, mentally, is only on page 8. When discussing the rationale, you want to first elicit *what* the client knows about the task and then elicit *why* it might be important (blending in the evoking process) using ATA. The client likely was introduced to the basics of the cognitive model in earlier sessions (e.g., during assessment, treatment planning, and possibly self-monitoring). Your first elicitation (*ask*) about what the client knows about managing thoughts should induce some recall about the links between situations, thoughts, emotions, and behaviors. Then you fill in the blanks (*tell*), and you elicit feedback (*ask*). In this way, you blend collaborative education with discussion of the rationale.

What information is useful during the "tell" component of this discussion? Leahy (2003) suggests addressing how thoughts create feelings and how thoughts are different from facts. Engaging the client can lay the groundwork for later focusing on identifying negative thoughts and evaluating them with evidence (collaborative empiricism). Using ATA, the discussion between you and your client should be about how thoughts create feelings using examples from previous discussions, hypothetical situations, or a worksheet. The idea is for the client to distinguish between thoughts and feelings so that later you can guide him or her to change thoughts as a way of increasing or decreasing a feeling. Traditional CBT proposes that thoughts are easier to change than feelings, and while feelings are uncontestable, thoughts are not. You may have previously discussed specific examples of thoughts that contribute to feelings, as in the case of Celia below. Note how the practitioner blends education with engaging Celia in a discussion of the rationale for the intervention strategy.

PRACTITIONER: What do you know so far about how thoughts affect feelings? [Ask]

CELIA: We talked last time about how situations, thoughts, and feelings are all related. Certain things trigger my feelings.

PRACTITIONER: You remember that these things are linked. [Reflect] So last time you told me about how the weather was bad, and you felt kind of low, that the weather made you feel even lower, and you just did not want to leave the house, so you called in sick to work. Then you felt guilty. If it's OK with you, let's figure out what were the thoughts and what were the feelings. You said you felt kind of low. That was a feeling. [Tell] What did you say to yourself that created that feeling? [Ask]

CELIA: Well, it's just that I have a lot I need to figure out at work, and I thought that if I went in I would just feel overwhelmed and not be able to do it. I can't stand the rain, and that made me feel like staying home and watching TV in bed instead. Plus, if I went in, and didn't finish everything, my boss would yell at me.

PRACTITIONER: OK, so let's write this down so we can really map it out. Some thoughts were (1) I have a lot I need to figure out at work, (2) if I go in I will feel overwhelmed and not be able to do it, (3) I hate the rain, and (4) if I don't finish everything, my boss will yell at me. [Reflect] The thoughts were about your ability to deal with the tasks at work. [Tell] What do you think the feelings were? [Ask]

CELIA: I'm not sure.

PRACTITIONER: It is hard to separate thoughts and feelings [Reflect], but, from a CBT model, which we have been talking about, thoughts are easier to examine, evaluate, and consider changing than feelings. If we can talk about the thoughts, then we can figure out how they affect the feelings. [Tell] What do you think of that approach? [Ask]

CELIA: I'm not sure. I have to see it to believe it.

PRACTITIONER: It is hard to imagine looking at your thoughts, potentially changing how you think about situations like this, and then feeling better, but you are willing to try it to see if it works for you. [Action reflection]

CELIA: OK . . .

PRACTITIONER: OK. So picture yourself back in that situation, thinking, "I have a lot I need to figure out at work, "If I go in I will feel overwhelmed and not be able to do it," "I hate the rain," and "If I don't finish everything, my boss will yell at me." What were you feeling, emotionally, when those thoughts were going through your head that morning.

CELIA: Overwhelmed and dread, I guess.

You and the client might discuss this as being a first step in learning to "restructure" one's thoughts when feeling negative emotions. Depending on the client and your judgment, you might identify a new or hypothetical situation and discuss how the same situation can yield different thoughts and then different feelings. You could then proceed to trying to label the thoughts or come up with a rational response.

PRACTITIONER: How would you feel about imagining a situation so we can explore the difference between thoughts and feelings? [Ask]

EUGENE: Sure.

PRACTITIONER: Imagine you go to your boyfriend's house and he grunts hello instead of giving you a kiss. You might think, "He is mad at me." What would you feel?

EUGENE: Upset and worried!

PRACTITIONER: If you thought he was mad at you, you would be upset and you would worry about it. [Reflect] What if you thought, "He must have had a really bad day at work," then what would you feel?

EUGENE: Well, depending on my mood, I would feel mad that he is taking it out on me or I might feel bad for him that he had a rough day.

PRACTITIONER: So in this case you would be more mad or sympathetic instead of upset or worried. [Reflect] Why do you think it might be important to figure out how thoughts create feelings? [Ask]

EUGENE: Well, I guess I need to find out why he didn't kiss me before I jump to conclusions.

PRACTITIONER: So checking out the facts to see if the thought is correct or not might be important. [Action reflection]

Returning to Celia, at this point, with permission, you might go back to restructuring the situation of that morning. You and your client can complete a worksheet recording what she thinks (or she says to herself) and then what she feels (using feelings words). Alternatively, there are worksheets you could use, with lists of thoughts and then a place to complete the feelings column, and vice versa (e.g., see *www.cci.health.wa.gov.au/docs/BB-3-The%20Thinking-Feeling%20Connection.pdf*).

A second piece of information alluded to in the example of Eugene is distinguishing thoughts from facts. Thoughts are hypotheses, descriptions, perspectives, and sometimes guesses. They can be true or false or partially true or false. At this point, you may not have engaged the client sufficiently to start challenging thoughts via Socratic questioning, but you can engage the client in the idea that distinguishing between thoughts and facts can be beneficial. Continuing the case of Eugene above, the practitioner elicits the rationale for distinguishing between thoughts and facts.

> PRACTITIONER: You explained really well how there could be different reasons for why your boyfriend did not greet you nicely. [Affirming reflection] So how would you find out these explanations? [Ask]
>
> EUGENE: I guess I could ask him before I reacted.
>
> PRACTITIONER: You would find out more information to check out the facts. [Reflect] You could then decide if your thought, "He must be mad at me," is true or false or partially true or false. [Tell and pause]
>
> EUGENE: Yeah, I usually don't check out the facts, I just get upset.
>
> PRACTITIONER: You can see how checking out the facts might help you from jumping to conclusions and being upset. [Reflect]
>
> EUGENE: Yeah, I just don't know how to do it.
>
> PRACTITIONER: So learning and practicing how to separate the facts from the thoughts could help with things like feeling upset. [Action reflection]

As before, you can consider hypothetical situations by identifying different thoughts in response to the same activating event. This can be done via dialogue or a worksheet (see Client Handout 5.1) where you list hypothetical events (e.g., It's raining) and then list two alternate beliefs or thoughts (e.g., I will get into an accident; I might need to drive slower to work) and the consequent feelings and behaviors (e.g., I feel scared and I will miss work; I will call if I am going to be late). Another strategy (see Client Handout 5.2) is to list different thoughts (e.g., he must be mad at me) and then several possible explanations for each thought (e.g., he had a bad day at work, I haven't done anything to make him mad). Again, you use ATA and discuss the rationale while filling in the gaps with education.

TIP for Engaging:
Personalized Feedback Using a Belief Rating

Either in session or using a self-monitoring log between sessions, ask the client to record situations and the associated thoughts. The client then rates the extent to which he or she believes the thought from 0 to 100%. Because clients inevitably vary the degree to which they believe certain thoughts, the variability demonstrates that thoughts are different than facts. For example, the client believes 95% that she cannot do anything right, but believes 80% that she is unlovable. Sometimes the belief rating varies by situation. For example, a client believes he can't do anything right. The client believes this 95% when he is with his spouse but only 20% when he is at the gym. These ratings can be presented back to the client using the personal feedback strategies described in Chapter 3.

Sustain Talk and Discord

In cognitive restructuring, the practitioner and the client together investigate the validity of the client's thoughts and beliefs, a process known as "collaborative empiricism." Gilbert and Leahy (2007) describe collaborative empiricism as a dance between two partners, where the practitioner and the client move together in time because both are sources of knowledge and experience. Miller and Rollnick (2012) describe sustain talk and discord as like wrestling instead of dancing. You can decrease sustain talk and prevent discord by eliciting the client's thoughts using ATA and attending to potential sustain talk (statements against cognitive restructuring) using the strategies described earlier (reflecting and emphasizing autonomy). Cognitive restructuring can elicit discord when clients feel invalidated, like their feelings are wrong or that their thoughts are always in error. This is why it is critically important, from an MI–CBT integrated approach, to be clear about the links between thoughts and feelings (feelings make sense in the context of certain thoughts) and that thoughts vary in their degree of "rightness." In fact it is a cognitive distortion to believe that thoughts are all right or all wrong. We prefer to avoid words like "errors" or "distortions" and instead prefer the term "unhelpful thoughts." This approach is similar to our earlier suggestion to avoid diagnostic terms or the word "problem." We want to avoid labeling and taking an expert stance and instead promote collaboration in a guiding style.

> Avoid words like "errors" or "distortions," and instead use the term "unhelpful thoughts."

> PRACTITIONER: I see you completed the first column in your automatic thought record when you were considering trying to start a conversation with the person who sits next to you in class.

SAM: Yes, that caused me a lot of anxiety.

PRACTITIONER: It was hard but you managed. [Affirming reflection] You wrote down "He will think I am a loser" as a thought, and then, for evidence, you wrote "Because my face will be red" and "Because I have no friends," but then I do not see any notation of what type of "unhelpful thought" it is, or a rational response.

SAM: Well, that is because I think both of those things are true.

PRACTITIONER: So, for you, both of these thoughts seem true. [Reflect] That's why we don't call them right thoughts or wrong thoughts, but rather helpful or unhelpful thoughts. So you said this thought makes you anxious and is unhelpful. Looking at this list, what do you think the thought "He will think I am a loser" corresponds to?

SAM: Labeling?

Focusing

The goal of the focusing process is to determine which unhelpful thoughts to address and to find the patterns among these thoughts. Finding the patterns allows the client to address categories of thoughts and to simplify the strategies for altering the thoughts and the consequent feelings and behaviors. You and your client can determine thoughts in session by analyzing different situations, as in the earlier examples, or you and your client may consider a thought record as a self-monitoring exercise. If the client is not able to identify automatic thoughts, you can ask the client's permission to visualize the concerning situation, role-play the situation, ask the client for the meaning of the situation, or offer a menu of helpful and unhelpful thoughts. In traditional CBT, the next step is to categorize the thoughts into specific cognitive distortions by going over a list of typical cognitive distortions (or "thinking errors," usually 10 or more). In MI–CBT, we are concerned about undermining the spirit of MI with an overly expert stance, lecturing the client at the risk of threatening engagement, and overwhelming the client with information and jargon. To avoid these traps, consider eliciting from the client potential patterns and together naming the pattern with a category that the client can connect to. As always, offer information or advice using ATA and a menu of options, as in the example below.

PRACTITIONER: Based on this thought record, there may be some similarities between your thoughts and the emotions they create. What do you notice about that? [Ask]

MARY: I feel depressed when I think bad things about myself.

PRACTITIONER: I see. And that can be difficult to manage. Let's look at this further: you notice that several unhelpful thoughts are about not liking yourself or thinking you are not good enough. [Reflect] Just looking at these thoughts and thinking about them, from this list here, what term could we use for this pattern so we can refer to it as we work on this? [Ask]

MARY: I don't know what you mean.

PRACTITIONER: Well, some people might call the pattern "all-or-nothing thinking" like you are all good or all bad. Some might call it "labeling" and another term could be "magnifying the negative." You could use one of these or you could call it something else so we can work on this pattern instead of each individual thought. [Tell with menu of options]

MARY: I guess labeling makes sense, or labeling the bad and ignoring the good.

PRACTITIONER: Labeling the bad makes a lot of sense and fits several of the thoughts you wrote down. [Reflect]

By the end of this process you will have guided your client to focus on his or her key thoughts and beliefs and elicited categories for the patterns as a way of emphasizing autonomy and paving the way for collaborative empiricism.

TIP for Focusing: Ensure Empathy

As you guide the client through the steps of cognitive restructuring, it is easy to get caught up in specific strategies and forget that the thoughts and feelings you are evaluating can be very painful. It is important to remember that you are a practitioner, not just a teacher, and that expressing empathy is a core component of maintaining the MI spirit and solidifying the therapeutic alliance in CBT. In addition to reflections, making supportive and compassionate statements about a difficult or painful situation, thought, or feeling expresses empathy and is critical to maintaining the alliance and the spirit of MI during the process of cognitive restructuring. The following dialogue picks up from the previous dialogue with Sam (from the "Engaging" section of this chapter) just after he has identified "labeling" as a description of his unhelpful thought that others will think he is a loser.

PRACTITIONER: Yes, that's right, you learn quickly. [Affirming reflection] Why might you think it is labeling. [Open question]

SAM: (*tearing up*) Because it is true. I am a loser. Only losers don't have any friends in college. I can't believe I am 19 years old, and can't make friends. . . . Just look at me and my life; this sucks.

PRACTITIONER: You are going through a really hard time right now. [Empathy with feelings reflection]

SAM: Yes, I mean I just don't like what is happening and I really want it to not be like this.

PRACTITIONER: You want your life to be different, and you've said that dealing with these distressing thoughts is one way to make it happen. [Reflection with action reflection]

SAM: Yes, that's it. I just wish it wasn't so hard.

PRACTITIONER: Yeah, it is really hard and you're very persistent. [Expressing empathy and affirming reflection]

Evoking

Recall that you evoke motivation by eliciting change language with certain types of questions. The goal is to guide the conversation so that the client verbalizes his or her own desire, ability, reasons, need, and commitment to change versus providing those statements for the client. In this way, the CBT strategy of guided inquiry using Socratic questioning can be highly consistent with an MI approach. "Socratic questioning" is a method originally developed by Socrates to stimulate critical thinking with questions instead of by providing information. Instead of offering evaluations or interpretations, the questions are meant to guide clients to evaluate their own thoughts. In MI–CBT, the process must be collaborative versus arrogant with a spirit of exploration versus that of renovation or fixing what is wrong (Miller, 1999). Padesky (1993) reminds practitioners that the purpose of Socratic questioning is guided discovery, not changing minds. She describes Socratic questions as those that the client has the knowledge to answer, that guide the client to consider relevant information that may be outside his or her current focus, that move from the concrete to the more abstract, and that support the client in applying the new information to arrive at a new conclusion.

The Foundation for Critical Thinking developed a taxonomy of Socratic questions (Paul & Elder, 2006) that have been adapted for CBT to evaluate thoughts (Beck, 2011). These include *questions about the evidence* for and against an unhelpful thought and questions about alternative explanations. *Decatastrophizing questions* guide the client to think about the worst thing that might happen and how the client would manage that worst-case scenario. *Impact questions* ask the client to hypothesize about the consequences of responding to the thought and the consequences of not responding. Finally, *questions to gain distance* from the thought guide the client to think about what he or she might tell a friend or family member in the same situation.

Padesky (1993) specifies three additional stages of Socratic questioning necessary for guided discovery: listening, summarizing, and asking synthesizing or analytical questions. MI specifies four skills to realize these stages: open questioning, reflective listening, summarizing, and asking a key question. In the case example below, Celia and the practitioner demonstrate guided discovery including all four stages using MI skills.

PRACTITIONER: You said one of the patterns on your log sheet is that you think that if you cannot finish everything at work, you will get yelled at by your boss. Let's go through this a bit further. What's the evidence that this will happen? [Evidence question]

CELIA: Sometimes he gives me mean looks, particularly when I am unsure about something.

PRACTITIONER: OK, so one piece of evidence for the prediction that he will yell at you is that he gives you mean looks sometimes. [Reflect] What other evidence do you have? [Evidence question]

CELIA: I have seen him snap at a coworker before.

PRACTITIONER: And so you think he might snap at you. [Reflect]

CELIA: I guess so, yes.

PRACTITIONER: So, two pieces of evidence are that he gives you mean looks sometimes, and that you have seen him snap before. [Reflect] What would be evidence that he might not yell at you? [Evidence question]

CELIA: I mean there is a lot of work to do, and he has said he knows this.

PRACTITIONER: So you have also seen him be understanding about the amount of work you have to do. [Reflect] What other evidence do you have that he might not yell at you? [Evidence question]

CELIA: Well, that other coworker that he snapped at was always late, never finishes his work, and leaves early. Everyone has to make up for his unfinished work, and we are all continually frustrated with him.

PRACTITIONER: I think I might be understanding this a bit better now. OK, so evidence against is that (1) he has been understanding to you, and (2) he snapped at the coworker who was having a lot of additional work problems. [Reflect] Do I have this right?

CELIA: Yes

PRACTITIONER: What kinds of things would you tell a friend who is worried about her boss yelling at her even though she is trying the best she can? [Distancing question]

CELIA: Well, I guess all I can do is try the best I can and hope he doesn't yell.

PRACTITIONER: Trying the best you can sounds good. [Reflect] What else might you say to a friend about this? [Alternative question]

CELIA: Well, if he does yell, it might not be about you as much as the overall situation.

PRACTITIONER: So when you have a lot on your plate at work, you worry you won't finish and your boss will yell at you. You have some evidence that he does snap at people sometimes when they don't finish their work. You said this is more of an issue when people tend to consistently not finish their work. Things like doing the best you can and thinking about alternative explanations if he does get angry might help. [Summarize] How does this information fit with your thought about having bad things happen at work? [Synthesizing/analytical question per Padesky or key question per MI]

CELIA: It's helping me think about other ways to think! I'm still not sure I can actually do it, but at least it makes sense.

Note that the last question the practitioner asks in this example begins to move from the concrete (boss will yell) to the more abstract (something bad will happen). Later you and the client can work toward developing general strategies (e.g., evidence questions) to address the pattern of thoughts (e.g., catastrophizing thoughts). While Celia's therapist has evoked the importance of changing thoughts, there are clearly still concerns about confidence based on Celia's last comment. This issue can be addressed with strategies to evoke confidence discussed in Chapter 2 (e.g., identifying personal strengths). Practicing skills in session, potentially via a role play, to manage thoughts as discussed below and in Chapter 6 is another way to build self-efficacy through a process of rehearsal and feedback.

Planning

In the other processes the client discussed *whether* and *why* to change thinking. In the planning process the discussion is about *how* to change thinking. These processes overlap significantly, do not need to occur sequentially, and may not even happen in the same session, but all the processes are relevant for cognitive restructuring. In the planning process you guide the client to make a plan for change, focusing on between-session activities (i.e., homework or practice), and consolidating commitment for that plan. The plan could include using Socratic questions to evaluate thoughts in between sessions and developing alternative thoughts and self-statements. These alternative thoughts and self-statements can be

Guide the client to make a plan for change, focusing on between-session activities and consolidating commitment.

developed in sessions, and role-play practice can increase confidence to manage thoughts between sessions (see Client Handout 5.3).

In addition to undergoing guided discovery by answering Socratic questioning, the client may plan to conduct behavioral experiments to test thoughts. A behavioral experiment for Mary might compare two approaches to overeating, "If I criticize myself when overeating, I'll overeat less" compared to "If I talk to myself kindly, I'll overeat less."? Mary might try each approach and monitor the consequences (e.g., food intake). This behavioral experiment might counteract a thought like "If I don't criticize myself, I will overeat and lose all self-control." After discussing the rationale and eliciting change talk for the experiment, you guide the client in the following steps: (1) identify the problem; (2) define the target thought; (3) consider an alternate perspective; (4) develop two possible hypotheses or predictions; and (5) plan for conducting the experiment. After the experiment the client will then discuss the outcome and how that influenced the target thought. A behavioral experiment form completed by Eugene is presented in Figure 5.1; a blank form is provided in Client Handout 5.4.

Step 1: What is my challenge?

I want to ask my boyfriend to remind me to take my medications, but I'm afraid to ask him for help.

Step 2: What is the main thought I have about my challenge?

He might be annoyed with me.

Step 3: What alternative perspective could I take?

He might want to help me.

Step 4: My predictions based on my main thought and alternative perspective

Main thought:	*Alternative perspective:*
He will yell at me and tell me that I should have figured it out a long time ago. He might decide that he doesn't want to be with me anymore.	*He'll say that he knows it's hard to remember and that he thought I didn't want help because I usually don't want to talk about it.*

Step 5: My plan to test my predictions

Ask him if he will help me when we go out to dinner on Wednesday and write down which prediction was as closest to what actually happens.

If this happens . . .	*Then I will . . .*
I might forget	*Set a reminder in my phone calendar*
I might have a few drinks and decide that I don't want to deal with it	*Talk to him in the car on the way to dinner*

FIGURE 5.1. Eugene's experiment.

See how the practitioner guides Eugene through these steps with MI skills.

PRACTITIONER: One of the things that you said might help you is if your boy-friend reminded you about your medications, but you are afraid to ask him for help. [Reflect; identify problem] Tell me more about that. [Open question]

EUGENE: I don't want him to get annoyed with me or think I am sick. And I don't want him to have to think about my status all the time.

PRACTITIONER: If you ask him for help, he might get annoyed with you and think badly of you. [Reflect; define target thought]

EUGENE: Yeah, I mean I hope not, but that's what stops me from getting him involved at all.

PRACTITIONER: You hope not, like there might be another way to think about it. [Reflect] What would be another way of seeing the situation, like another perspective about how your boyfriend might react? [Consider an alternate perspective]

EUGENE: Sometimes I think he might want to help me. Maybe he doesn't know how. Or maybe he avoids it because I don't want to think about it.

PRACTITIONER: So you have two possible predictions about what might hap-pen if you ask for help. One—he might be annoyed with you. Two—he might want to help you. [Reflect; develop alternative hypotheses or pre-dictions] So what could you do this week to test these two possibilities?

EUGENE: Ask him for help?

PRACTITIONER: You could ask him for help and record which of these two predictions was more accurate. [Reflect; plan for conducting the experi-ment] When would you plan to do this?

EUGENE: I'm not sure. We are going out to dinner on Wednesday.

PRACTITIONER: You already have a time and place in mind to conduct this "experiment." [Affirm] What might get in the way? [Develop if–then plans]

EUGENE: I don't know. I might forget, or if we have a few drinks I might not want to deal with it.

PRACTITIONER: So forgetting or avoiding are the two barriers. [Reflect] How could you handle the remembering to ask him? [Open question]

EUGENE: I don't think that's really a problem because I can plan to talk to him around our dinner date, but I can put a reminder in my phone calendar.

PRACTITIONER: OK, you can put that reminder in right now if you want. What about the avoiding part? [Open question]

EUGENE: I'm not sure. What do you think?

PRACTITIONER: Some people try telling the person ahead of time that they have something to talk about at dinner so that they don't avoid it. Another choice is to practice here so that you know exactly how it goes or you can try to ask him on your way to dinner before you have a drink. It's up to you. [Menu of options; emphasize autonomy]

EUGENE: I don't feel like practicing now, and if I tell him ahead of time it's like making a big deal. But I can do it in the car on the way to dinner.

One thing to consider here is that Eugene's boyfriend could be annoyed if Eugene asks him for help taking his medicines. It is important to plan for different outcomes in these types of cognitive-behavioral experiments. You might explore with Eugene what his reaction would be if his boyfriend is willing to help, and if he is not willing to help and is annoyed. This might involve a full-length cognitive restructuring activity specifically about thoughts like "If he is annoyed with me that would mean that I am 'less than as a person for needing to be on medicines' or 'I can't take care of myself without another person.' "

Another possible plan might be graduated exposure, the systematic confrontation of feared internal (thoughts, physical reactions) or external (activities, situations) stimuli. While a full discussion of exposure therapy is beyond the scope of this chapter, you may consider adapting the discussion on behavioral experiments to include exposure activity as an experiment where the client is testing his or her response to stimuli of increasing intensity. Other approaches such as relaxation training and acceptance or mindfulness are discussed in Chapter 6.

Once the client has developed a plan for change, recall that you consolidate commitment by (1) developing action steps including implementation intentions (when–then plans); (2) identifying potential barriers to implementation; (3) generating solutions to potential barriers (if–then plans); and (4) reinforcing commitment with open questions to elicit commitment language, scaling questions or rulers, affirming reflections, and expressions of hope and optimism. Chapters 2, 3, and 4 provide more detail about these components of the planning process. See Client Handout 5.5 for a Change Plan form for cognitive restructuring and Figure 5.2 for a sample Change Plan for Sam.

MI–CBT Dilemmas

As in self-monitoring, the key dilemma when guiding a client in cognitive restructuring is how to manage when the client is not ready to engage in cognitive restructuring and you believe it is a critical ingredient for successful treatment. Again, you have choices. You may inform the client that cognitive restructuring is necessary

My Plan for Thinking Skills

Changes I would like to make:

Learn to manage my social anxiety

These changes are important to me because:

I do not want to feel lonely or depressed.

I want to make some friends.

I want to have a girlfriend.

I want to enjoy being in college.

I do not want to avoid taking classes if I have to give a presentation.

How thinking skills can help me:

I can find different ways to think, which help me feel better.

If I feel better, then I might be able to get more things I want like a girlfriend
or better grades.

I plan to do these thinking skills (what, where, when, how):

1. Try to ignore unhelpful "stuck" thoughts about social situations with peers.
2. Replace unhelpful "stuck" thoughts with more helpful thoughts from my thought
   log, which I will complete every day. I will keep the log by my bed, and take a
   picture of it on my phone.
3. Try mindfulness practice if steps 1 and 2 don't work.
4. Discuss differences in my next session and make a plan to use the most successful
   strategy.

IF this gets in the way	THEN try this
I cannot ignore my thoughts.	Practice focusing on the more helpful thoughts with therapist in next session.
	Notice that the thought is there, that I cannot control if a particular thought is in my head, but then try to focus on the more helpful thoughts instead.
I don't have my thought log sheet with me.	Take a photo of sheet on my phone.

FIGURE 5.2. Sam's Change Plan for cognitive skills.

for the CBT you provide and that if the client is not ready to complete the task, then he or she may not be ready for CBT. Alternatively, you can decide to provide MI–CBT without cognitive restructuring, perhaps asking the client to revisit the idea if progress is not sufficient. Finally, you may provide a menu of options that includes cognitive restructuring but also other options such as mindfulness, acceptance, and commitment therapy strategies, and problem-solving approaches.

Another dilemma concerns traditional CBT's view of automatic thoughts as one level of cognitions with beliefs, particularly core beliefs, at a deeper level that requires restructuring. Schema therapy is an example of an approach that addresses deeply held beliefs and patterns of thought (Farrell, Reiss, & Shaw, 2014). In MI–CBT, if symptoms begin to resolve by evaluating and replacing automatic thoughts and patterns of thoughts, it may not be necessary to dig down to uncover core beliefs. Furthermore, if core beliefs are tied to core values, you may encounter significant difficulty (sustain talk and discord) by addressing core beliefs. This is another choice point for you as the practitioner. You can continue to address core beliefs or you can move onto other strategies to guide the client to resolve concerns. Finally, as can be seen in Eugene's case above, the client may choose to avoid practicing in session. This is a dilemma if you consider a core element of CBT to be practice within as well as between sessions. We recommend exploring ambivalence around practicing including eliciting the rationale, but supporting the client's autonomy to not practice. Consider practicing the next session if the client struggles during the week.

ACTIVITY 5.1 FOR PRACTITIONERS

Open-Ended Socratic Questions

Socratic questions guide the client to evaluate his or her own thoughts. In MI–CBT, the spirit should be collaborative and exploratory versus expert renovation. Using open-ended versus closed-ended questions promotes this spirit.

ACTIVITY GOAL: In this activity you will integrate MI and CBT by converting Socratic questions that are closed-ended into open-ended questions to guide cognitive change.

ACTIVITY INSTRUCTIONS: We provide several examples of closed-ended Socratic questions. Rewrite each into an open-ended question with the same function.

Sample

Closed ended: Could you put that another way?

Open ended: *How would you put that another way?*

You Try!

1. Closed ended: Is this good evidence for believing that?

   Open ended: _____

2. Are those reasons good enough?

   Open ended: _____

3. Is there reason to doubt that evidence?

   Open ended: _____

4. Did anyone else see this another way?

   Open ended: _____

5. Do we need facts to answer this?

   Open ended: _____

6. Is there a more logical explanation?

   Open ended: _____

7. Is this the only explanation?

   Open ended: _____

8. Have you always felt this way?

   Open ended: _____

9. Do you think that will work?

   Open ended: _____

10. Anything else?

   Open ended: _____

ACTIVITY 5.2 FOR PRACTITIONERS

Sequences: Eliciting and Reinforcing Change Talk for Cognitive Restructuring

ACTIVITY GOAL: In this activity you will practice developing evoking questions to elicit change talk specifically for cognitive restructuring. You will then develop a reflection to reinforce the change talk.

ACTIVITY INSTRUCTIONS: For each of the following items, fill in the blanks, making up additional details of the case as necessary. You will practice completing each of the three components of the sequences. In the first section, you will complete one of the three components of the sequence (question to elicit change talk, client change talk, reflection of change talk). In the second section, you will use your creativity to complete two of the three components.

Item 1

- **Practitioner Strategy to Elicit Change Talk:** What evidence is there that you always drink when you get together with your family?
- **Client Change Talk:** It's just what we do. I go to someone's house and they put a beer in my hand. If I say "No," then it's, "C'mon . . . just one! Lighten up!" And then it's one more, and one more. That's just how it is.
- **Practitioner Reinforcement (Reflection/Question):** _____
  _____
  _____

Item 2

- **Practitioner Strategy to Elicit Change Talk:** What evidence is there that you can get together with them and not drink?
- **Client Change Talk:** _____
  _____
  _____
- **Practitioner Reinforcement (Reflection/Question):** Being in a different situation, like with the kids at the zoo, took the pressure off.

Item 3

- **Practitioner Strategy to Elicit Change Talk:** _____
  _____
  _____
- **Client Change Talk:** I'd say it's all about choices. You don't have to stop being with the people who are important to you, but you can choose the situations. Choose the ones that aren't drinking situations and it'll be easier. I guess that's what I need to do too.
- **Practitioner Reinforcement (Reflection/Question):** You don't have to give up what's important to you, and you can choose to do things that put your goals in reach. Choices.

Item 4

- **Practitioner Strategy to Elicit Change Talk:** Sam, now that we've talked about some of the things that are important to you, like making friends and fitting in, I'd like to ask you what happens when you have thoughts like "I'll never have any friends"?
- **Client Change Talk:** _____
  _____
  _____
- **Practitioner Reinforcement (Reflection/Question):** _____
  _____
  _____

Item 5

- **Practitioner Strategy to Elicit Change Talk:** _____
  _____
  _____

- **Client Change Talk:** I guess, if I didn't have so many stuck thoughts, then I could probably ignore them and do something . . . talk to someone who wouldn't judge me, or go somewhere and not worry about what it means if I don't fit in. . . . I guess that's what people do if they're not like me.

- **Practitioner Reinforcement (Reflection/Question):** _____
  _____
  _____

Item 6

- **Practitioner Strategy to Elicit Change Talk:** _____
  _____
  _____

- **Client Change Talk:** _____
  _____
  _____

- **Practitioner Reinforcement (Reflection/Question):** Being able to ignore them sometimes could help you to start some friendships.

Suggested Responses

Item 1

- **Practitioner Reinforcement (Reflection/Question):** You feel like you can't get away from it. Like it's an expectation.

Item 2

- **Client Change Talk:** I guess I have done things with my family that don't involve drinking. It's a big part of what we do, but . . . well, a few of us got together over the summer and took the kids to the zoo.

Item 3

- **Practitioner Strategy to Elicit Change Talk:** Given that, if you had a friend who was having a hard time—he wanted to stop drinking, but didn't want to stop seeing his family—what advice would you give him?

Item 4

- **Client Change Talk:** Nothing. It feels like nothing will ever change and there isn't anything I can do about it. I just think about how much I wish I could fix it.
- **Practitioner Reinforcement (Reflection/Question):** You end up feeling stuck, but if there was something you could do, then you'd want to do it.

Item 5

- **Practitioner Strategy to Elicit Change Talk:** How do you think things might be different if you didn't have those stuck thoughts?
- **Practitioner Reinforcement (Reflection/Question):** You're wondering if people who go out and do some of the things that you want to do either don't have stuck thoughts, or they can ignore them.

Item 6

- **Practitioner Strategy to Elicit Change Talk:** What do you think would happen if you could ignore those thoughts too?
- **Client Change Talk:** I don't know if I could ignore them all the time, but if I could do it sometimes, then I might be able to talk to other people enough to start making some friends.

Situations, Thoughts, Feelings, and Behaviors

Situations lead to you thinking, feeling, or behaving a certain way, but there is more than one way to think or feel for each situation. For example, some people think that if they have to speak in public, they will make a fool of themselves, so they skip class. Other people might think that if they have to speak in public, they need to be more prepared to study harder. Consider and write down different situations that lead you to think, feel, or behave a certain way and then consider other thoughts, feelings, or behaviors for that situation.

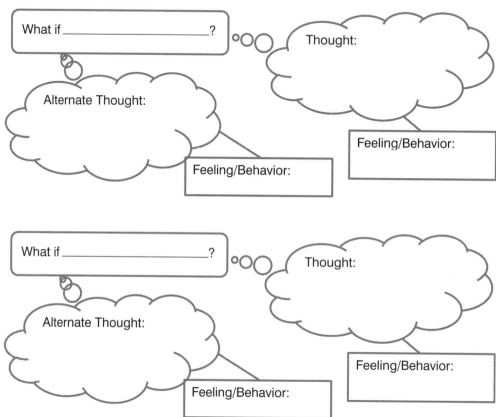

SITUATIONS AND ALTERNATE EXPLANATIONS

List three reasons why you choose to complete this worksheet:

1. _____

2. _____

3. _____

Situations and Alternate Explanations

People interpret situations in different ways, but most situations have more than one interpretation. You may typically interpret a situation in a way that makes you feel badly, but you can also consider alternative explanations. For example, your partner is short with you when he comes home from work. You might think that he is irritated by you, and you feel rejected. However, what are some alternative explanations? He may have had a bad day at work, or perhaps the traffic coming home was terrible. These alternative explanations might lead you to feel less rejected. Why would you want to consider practicing alternative explanations: _____

_____

_____

_____.

Situation	Your Usual Explanation	One Alternative Explanation	Another Alternative Explanation
Example: My partner is short with me.	*Example:* I'm irritating him.	*Example:* He had a hard day at work.	*Example:* He got stuck in traffic.

Helpful and Unhelpful Thoughts

Write *unhelpful* thoughts that you sometimes have, then practice turning them into *helpful* thoughts.

Why would it be helpful to *you* to practice turning unhelpful thoughts into more helpful thoughts?

How could you see yourself doing this when you have an unhelpful thought?

Unhelpful Thoughts	Helpful Thoughts
Example: *I can't do anything right.*	Example: *Sometimes I make mistakes, but I do a lot of things right.*

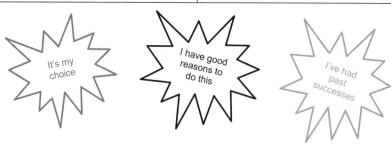

It's my choice

I have good reasons to do this

I've had past successes

Behavioral Experiments

A behavioral experiment can be used to test your thoughts about what might happen if you take alternative actions when faced with one of your challenges. See the example below, then fill out your own behavioral experiment form.

Sample:

Step 1: What is my challenge?
I want to ask my boyfriend to remind me to take my medications, but I'm afraid to ask him for help.

Step 2: What is the main thought I have about my challenge?
He might be annoyed with me.

Step 3: What alternative perspective could I take?
He might want to help me.

Step 4: My predictions based on my main thought and alternative perspective

Main thought:	*Alternative perspective:*
He will yell at me and tell me that I should have figured it out a long time ago. He might decide that he doesn't want to be with me anymore.	*He'll say that he knows it's hard to remember and that he thought I didn't want help because I usually don't want to talk about it.*

Step 5: My plan to test my predictions

Ask him if he will help me when we go out to dinner on Wednesday and write down which prediction is closest to what actually happens.

If this happens . . .	*Then I will . . .*
I might forget.	*Set a reminder in my phone calendar.*
I might have a few drinks and decide that I don't want to deal with it.	*Talk to him in the car on the way to dinner.*

Complete this form with your practitioner to test your thoughts about what might happen if you take alternative actions when faced with one of your challenges.

(continued)

MY EXPERIMENT

Why would you want to test to see how accurate your thoughts are or whether there is another perspective instead: _____

Step 1: What is my challenge?

Step 2: What is the main thought I have about my challenge?

Step 3: What alternative perspective could I take?

Step 4: My predictions based on my main thought and alternative perspective
Main thought: *Alternative perspective:*

Step 5: My plan to test my predictions
.
If this happens . . .   *Then I will . . .*

What happened? _____

_____

_____

What will you do the next time you have this kind of situation? _____

_____

_____

Change Plan for Cognitive Skills

My Plan for Thinking Skills

Changes I would like to make:

_____

_____

_____

_____

These changes are important to me because:

_____

_____

_____

_____

How thinking skills can help me:

_____

_____

_____

_____

I plan to take these steps for thinking skills (what, where, when, how):

_____

_____

_____

_____

IF this gets in the way   **THEN try this**

_____   _____

_____   _____

_____   _____

_____   _____

_____   _____

CHAPTER 6

Behavioral and Emotion Regulation Skills

While there are numerous behavioral and emotion regulation skills under the umbrella of CBT, we focus our discussion on those most commonly referenced in CBT and those that are most relevant to our case concerns—alcohol use, depression, anxiety, medical conditions, and obesity. These include problem-solving skills, behavioral activation, distress tolerance, mindfulness, exposure therapy, stimulus control of worry, and assertiveness training. We first briefly describe each skill for practitioners less familiar with skills training.

Problem-Solving Skills

Problem-solving skills are utilized in many CBT approaches that focus on identifying triggers and developing coping strategies. Problem-solving skills training has the following components. First, the client learns to develop a positive problem orientation with education and possibly the cognitive skills described in the previous chapter. This means reframing a problem as a solvable challenge and increasing the client's belief that he or she can, in fact, manage it effectively with time and effort (see "Building Confidence" below). While no solution is easy or perfect, the idea is to make an informed choice as to the best possible solution. You then help your client develop a rational problem-solving style with four major skill steps (see Client Handout 6.1): (1) formulating the problem; (2) generating (brainstorming) solutions; (3) making a decision based on evaluation of potential solutions; and (4) implementing the solution and analyzing its effect. When the client has chosen a solution, help break it down into manageable steps. Meta-analyses suggest that problem-solving skills training is effective across a variety of physical and mental health concerns and is most effective when all of the components are delivered (Bell & D'Zurilla, 2009).

Behavioral Activation

Behavioral activation was developed as a treatment for depression that focuses on context, such as increasing pleasurable and rewarding activities, rather than on internal processes, such as cognitions (Martell et al., 2010). From the behavioral activation perspective, depressive symptoms are viewed as a natural reaction to an environment with few positive reinforcers for activation and many negative reinforcers for avoidance behaviors. More recently, behavioral activation has been recommended for its ability to improve avoidance behaviors in anxiety as well (Chen, Liu, Rapee, & Pillay, 2013; Turner & Leach, 2009). Behavioral activation typically includes self-monitoring to identify the links between activities and mood (see Chapter 4). Then clients are asked to engage in activities (graded from simple to more complex) based on a goal or plan, and not based on their mood (see Client Handout 6.2). Typically, doing the activity comes first and feeling better comes a bit later. Some therapists use the phrase "Fake it until you make it" as a way to get their clients to start the treatment, with the promise that after doing it for a certain time, they will start to feel better. Clients' activity is monitored via daily mood and activity logs.

Every session is focused on what clients do, not on what they think, with special emphasis on activities that are naturally reinforcing (e.g., exercising, eating, socializing). Behavioral activation has received strong empirical support as a stand-alone treatment for depression (Mazzucchelli, Kane, & Rees, 2009; Sturmey, 2009). In their seminal study, Jacobson and colleagues (1996) showed that the behavioral activation component of CBT was as effective in the treatment of depression as a full CBT package.

A more recent replication of the Jacobson et al. (1996) study showed again that behavioral activation was as effective as traditional CBT in the treatment of depression, and that it was actually more effective than CBT for participants who were rated as being more "severely depressed" (Dimidjian et al., 2006). Importantly, these findings have suggested that targeting overt behavior change alone was sufficient to produce corresponding improvements in covert correlates of depression (i.e., thinking and feeling).

Distress Tolerance

Several named treatments considered under the umbrella of CBT, including dialectical behavior therapy (Dimeff & Koerner, 2007) and affect regulation training

(Berking & Whitley, 2014), address emotion regulation such as distress tolerance skills. "Distress tolerance" has been defined as the perceived ability to endure negative emotional states or the capacity to continue goal-directed behavior in the context of negative affect. The inability (or perceived inability) to tolerate distress has been associated with many psychological symptoms (Leyro, Zvolensky, & Bernstein, 2010) and physical health concerns such as depression and anxiety (Zvolensky, Vujanovic, Bernstein, & Leyro, 2010), medication adherence (Oser, Trafton, Lejuez, & Bonn-Miller, 2013), and overeating (Kozak & Fought, 2011). Berking and Whitley (2014) synthesized previous theories and delineated the skills necessary for emotion regulation: awareness, identification, correct interpretation of emotion–body sensations, understanding triggers, active modification of distress or acceptance and tolerance when modification is not possible, and confrontation versus avoidance of distressing situations (see Client Handouts 6.3 and 6.4). Note that in the cases of substance abuse and obesity, distress can take the form of cravings and hunger, and the strategies to manage distress are the same.

Strategies to help with distress include distraction, thinking about something else to allow the situation to "sit on the back burner," triggering other physical sensations (e.g., taking a cold shower, eating spicy food, exercising), and utilizing techniques such as relaxation. More recently, a strategy used to tolerate distress is mindfulness—nonjudgmental awareness of the moment. Learning mindfulness means experiencing distress but not adding to it by being upset about the distress. It involves learning that distress is part of life, and in reaction to it one can have thoughts like this: "This is what it feels like to be distressed. I can handle this. It is OK that I am feeling so upset right now." The idea is to learn, gradually, how to experience negative events and experiences for what they are in the moment.

Mindfulness

Mindfulness skills focus on increasing awareness of thoughts and feelings and learning to accept them without judgment and without attaching or reacting to them. Mindfulness can be considered an adjunct to distress tolerance, as the goal is mindful observation of thoughts, feelings, and sensations. This goal is often achieved with techniques like meditation, breathing exercises, and yoga. These approaches promote nonjudgmental awareness of life events and internal responses to them (mindfulness), rather than focusing on challenging the content of thoughts or emotions regarding stressful events. Mindfulness treatment approaches such as mindfulness-based CBT and mindfulness-based stress reduction have been shown to improve stress responses, psychological symptoms such as depression and anxiety, physical symptoms, substance use, and quality of life (Chiesa, Calati, & Serretti, 2011; Chiesa & Serretti, 2009; Fjorback, Arendt, Ørnbøl, Fink, & Walach, 2011).

Exposure Therapy

In exposure therapy, developed from the classical conditioning literature, clients make contact with a feared stimulus (real or imagined) until the associated anxiety diminishes. Some consider this process a form of learning how to better tolerate distress. This is the case for panic disorder, in that clients learn to be less anxious about the experience of anxiety. For other anxiety disorders, exposure requires that situations causing anxiety be tolerated until the anxiety diminishes. This can occur in a systematic way, starting with the creation of a fear hierarchy. The hierarchy is developed by the client rating fear situations from lowest to highest; a self-monitoring task can be used to facilitate these ratings (see Chapter 4). The client then undergoes exposures (*in vivo*—in real life—or in imagination) beginning with the least feared stimulus and then gradually moves up the fear hierarchy (see Figure 6.1 on page 136 for a sample fear hierarchy for Sam's social phobia).

Alternatively, in "flooding" (real exposure to the worst fear), the client faces the fear highest in the hierarchy. Most clinicians and patients prefer graduated exposure due to the discomfort of flooding (Öst, Alm, Brandberg, & Breitholtz, 2001; Moulds & Nixon, 2006), but in MI–CBT you would give the client this choice. Typically, clients are taught skills described above (e.g., distraction, relaxation, mindfulness) to cope with the distressing feelings that occur during exposure (see Client Handout 6.5). Meta-analysis of 20 trials suggested that cognitive restructuring and exposure have equivalent efficacy for most anxiety disorders (Ourgrin, 2011), and that virtual exposure therapy has equivalent efficacy to *in vivo* exposure (Powers & Emmelkamp, 2008).

Stimulus Control of Worry

"Worry" is an anxious preoccupation with an anticipated negative event. It is an effective short-term response to uncertainty, stimulating healthy attention and problem solving, but sometimes worrying can become self-perpetuating, be excessive, and have adverse long-term consequences. Excessive worry is a primary symptom of generalized anxiety disorder. Stimulus control for worry was originally proposed in the early 1980s (Borkovec, Wilkinson, Folensbee, & Lerman, 1983) and has received recent attention in clinical studies (McGowan & Behar, 2013; Verkuil, Brosschot, Korrelboom, Reul-Verlaan, & Thayer, 2011). The goal of stimulus control training is to limit how much time is spent worrying and to gradually associate worry with more distinct and specific times and locations. Only those times and locations come to elicit worry. The client is asked to identify a 30-minute "worry period" to occur at the same time and place each day but that is at least 3 hours before bedtime. The client is instructed to worry as intensely as possible during the 30-minute period, but the rest of the day he or she is supposed

		Fear rating (1–100)	Avoidance (1–100)
1	Going to a party (at school)	100	100
2	Starting a conversation with a girl I am attracted to	99	100
3	Attending a family event (like wedding or funeral or Thanksgiving)	70	40
4	Hanging out in the cafeteria or student union	65	70
5	Talking to the pharmacist or people in a store	60	60
6	Asking a professor for help	55	55
7	Sitting in a coffee shop	55	70
8	Maintaining a conversation with a male classmate when he starts the conversation	50	30
9	Going to the library	40	35
10	Being in class	40	5

```
0    10   20   30   40   50   60   70   80   90   100
+----+----+----+----+----+----+----+----+----+----+
No              Mild           Moderate      Severe      Very severe
anxiety/        anxiety/       anxiety/      anxiety/    anxiety/
avoidance       avoidance      avoidance     avoidance   avoidance
```

FIGURE 6.1. Sam's fear hierarchy.

to postpone any worry to the worry period and focus on the present moment (see Client Handout 6.6). Worry control is often included as part of anxiety treatment (Craske & Barlow, 2006). Moreover, recent pilot studies suggest that stimulus control alone may be superior to acceptance training on measures of worry and insomnia, and that worry control can enhance the effects of stress management training (McGowan & Behar, 2013; Verkuil et al., 2011).

Refusal Skills and Assertiveness Training

Refusal skills are included in several evidence-based approaches to treating addictive behaviors including behavioral self-control training (Walters, 2001).

Meta-analysis has shown refusal skills with assertiveness training to be a core component of effective substance abuse treatment (Magill, 2009) with refusal skills associated with better substance use outcomes compared to other CBT modules (Witkiewitz, Lustyk, & Bowen, 2013). Assertiveness training is also a key component of behavioral interventions for obesity (Jacob & Isaac, 2012).

There are two core components to refusal skills (see Client Handout 6.7). The first component involves avoiding situations in which triggers, including social pressure, are likely to occur. This component has also been called "environmental control," in which clients address ways to avoid triggers and to maximize facilitators of alternative behaviors. If the client cannot or chooses not to avoid situations, then the second component involves developing coping strategies for being exposed to triggers. These include assertive communication to address direct and indirect social pressure and an escape plan if the situation becomes too difficult to manage. Key components of assertive communication involve understanding the differences between assertive, aggressive, and passive language, and the utilization of "I" statements to describe one's feelings or reactions, followed by a specific request.

Additional Skills

There are many other skills available in the CBT literature that may be relevant for coping plans including communication skills (McHugh, Hearon, & Otto, 2010), social skills (Kurtz & Mueser, 2008; Monti & O'Leary, 1999), and organization and planning skills (Barkley, 2015; Lorig et al., 2001; Safren, Perlman, Sprich, & Otto, 2005). These skills may be all addressed with MI as a foundation for the four processes describe below.

Engaging

As described in earlier chapters, the engaging process incorporates checking in with a client about the previous week, using reflections, questions, and expressions of empathy to reinforce the therapeutic alliance and engagement in treatment. Furthermore, the beginning of each session includes reviewing components of the previous session, which at this point usually will include between-session practice. As in the case of cognitive skills, engaging includes collaborative agenda setting. The agenda can include behavioral or emotional regulation skills because they were prioritized as part of the initial treatment plan or because you and the client determined that these skills are useful based on reports from the previous week.

The next step is to discuss the rationale in general terms, waiting to discuss and evoke motivation for the specific details of the skills training until there is sufficient engagement around the session tasks. Refraining from problem solving until the planning process is critical because the goal of engaging is to listen and understand (avoid the "righting reflex"; be collaborative not prescriptive). Recall that when discussing the rationale, you want to first elicit *what* the client knows about the task and then elicit *why* it might be important (blending in the evoking process here) using ATA. Then you provide information (*tell*), and you elicit feedback (*ask*). In this way, you begin education with discussion of the rationale in an MI style.

> PRACTITIONER: One of the things that we talked about that could help you with figuring out how to manage tempting situations is problem-solving skills. What do you know about problem-solving skills? [Ask]
>
> MARY: Well, it's about how to figure out solutions to problems, but I don't know how to do it.
>
> PRACTITIONER: Right, learning problem-solving skills is a step-by-step process where you first brainstorm all possible solutions, then you look at the pros and cons of each, then you pick a solution to try. When that is done, you break down the solution into manageable steps. [Tell] Why do you think that would that be helpful? [Ask]
>
> MARY: I need to figure out how to deal with people who don't know how to help me when I'm trying to lose weight.
>
> PRACTITIONER: So for you, learning problem-solving skills will help you deal with people in your life. [Reflect]

Note how the same practitioner statements can be used for a different skill.

> PRACTITIONER: You said that you might be interested in learning some ways to handle distress when you think about your HIV status. One of the ways you can do this is with mindfulness. What have you heard about mindfulness, if anything? [Ask]
>
> EUGENE: Not much, but I think it is like meditation.
>
> PRACTITIONER: Right, it is like meditation. Mindfulness is about learning how to be aware of thoughts and feelings and how to accept them instead of react to them. Meditation is one way to do this. [Tell] Why would that be helpful? [Ask]
>
> EUGENE: I definitely need to learn to control my reactions.
>
> PRACTITIONER: So controlling your reactions to upsetting thoughts and feelings would help you cope, and learning mindfulness is one way to do this. [Reflect]

TIP for Engaging with Some Focusing:
Mini-Functional Analysis

As discussed in Chapter 3, the purpose of a functional analysis is to understand the function—the antecedents and consequences (e.g., places, time of day)—of the target behavior. At the beginning of treatment, the functional analysis focused on the presenting concerns. When reviewing the change plan, some practitioners prefer to begin each session with a short functional analysis of the progress or lack of progress in behavior change in the previous week. In this way, you may guide the client to refocus on skills from the original treatment plan or to develop a new focus on new skills relevant to current concerns. When integrating MI and CBT, MI skills such as using open-ended questions and balancing them with reflections and summaries ensure that the assessment remains collaborative (see Chapter 3). You can further build motivation for skills training by reinforcing any change talk tied to skills use.

PRACTITIONER: You mentioned that you had trouble last week at your nephew's birthday party.

CARL: Yes, in my family birthday parties are a chance for the adults to have fun together, which means drinking.

PRACTITIONER: Part of how your family celebrates is with alcohol. [Reflect]

CARL: Yeah. It's just what we do.

PRACTITIONER: Family events are a trigger for you, and it is really hard to say no in those situations. [Reflect]

CARL: Almost impossible.

PRACTITIONER: It feels almost impossible to say no in those situations, so figuring out how to refuse alcohol when your family gets together might be helpful to discuss today. [Action reflection]

CARL: Yeah, I've got to figure out something before the holidays coming up.

PRACTITIONER: Communicating to your family about drinking is something you need to work on and pretty quickly. [Reflection of change talk]

Focusing

The focusing process further clarifies the direction of treatment. While engaging includes collaboratively setting the agenda on which skills to address, focusing involves guiding the client to clarify which specific skill components in which contexts will be learned and practiced. Often, the client will need education about the skill in order to understand how it can be applied in his or her specific situation. In MI–CBT, education is provided using ATA and is followed by questions to focus the client on particular scenarios for practicing inside and outside of the session, as in the following example.

> Focusing involves guiding the client to clarify which specific skill components in which contexts will be learned and practiced.

PRACTITIONER: Before we talked about how there are some activities that make you feel better, less depressed. What do you remember about that? [Ask]

CELIA: Yeah, when I wrote down my activities for the day it seemed like I felt a little better when I was making dinner and worse when I was sitting around having a hard time deciding what to do.

PRACTITIONER: So cooking is one thing that improves your mood. [Reflect] One way of making your mood better is by planning activities that might make you feel better, and sticking to that plan even if it is harder than usual because you are not feeling well. [Tell] What do you think of that idea? [Ask]

CELIA: Certain things make me feel better but I don't know where to start.

PRACTITIONER: So you have some ideas about activities that might improve your mood but it feels overwhelming. [Reflect] One way to handle that is to take something you like to do and break it down into steps. Then you can plan activities step by step. [Tell] How do you think that would work? [Ask]

CELIA: We could try it.

PRACTITIONER: You're willing to give it a shot. [Reflect] Take cooking a special meal. What would be some steps to consider? [Ask]

CELIA: Well, I have to find a recipe, and then go grocery shopping.

PRACTITIONER: So a plan might look like tomorrow you find a recipe, Wednesday you grocery shop, and then Thursday you cook the special meal. [Tell] What other activities do you want to consider? [Ask]

CELIA: I think I like the cooking idea for now.

Evoking

Evoking motivation is about evoking importance (desire, reasons, or needs) and confidence (ability). The previous chapters have described strategies to evoke importance and confidence using open questions, rulers, affirming reflections, and identifying personal strengths. In order to promote adherence to CBT, it is critical not to skip this process and prematurely move to planning when the client has focused on specific skills. Bandura (2004) suggests additional strategies to promote self-efficacy for behavioral skills using role-play practice. These strategies include modeling, rehearsal (verbal/behavioral), and feedback (Miltenberger, 2008). After you model the skills step by step, the client then performs the steps while verbally stating each step (behavioral rehearsal). If this process is premature, the client can state the steps while you perform the skill (verbal rehearsal). MI skills may be necessary to address client concerns about role-play practice, and as always you must first elicit the rationale for this type of training. Feedback is given in a "sandwich" with something positive, something to improve on, and strengths the client has to support implementing this skill (see Client Handout 6.8).

> PRACTITIONER: So now that you have decided to use mindfulness to help your response to stressful situations, you want to start with when you lay in bed at night and can't sleep. Why do you think it would be helpful to practice this skill in the session? [Ask]
>
> EUGENE: I don't know how to do it, and reading instructions doesn't usually work for me.
>
> PRACTITIONER: Reading how to do it doesn't work as well as actually practicing it. [Reflect] It might be helpful for me to show the steps first. Then you can try them and I can give you feedback. If you say the steps out loud when you do them, it might help you remember them. [Tell] What do you think about that approach? [Ask]
>
> EUGENE: I guess anything to help me remember.

After the modeling and rehearsal, the practitioner gives feedback in an MI style including the following steps: solicit feedback from the client on his or her perceptions of what was done well and what he or she would like to improve; affirm correct steps; and offer suggestions for improvement.

> PRACTITIONER: You worked hard on that. [Affirm] How did you think it went? [Ask]
>
> MARY: I don't know. I mean it felt kind of silly singing to make me feel better but it kind of worked.
>
> PRACTITIONER: It felt silly, but you felt better. [Reflect] You identified that fights with your mom were a trigger for eating. You identified your warning signs and angry feelings. You practiced stepping away from the

kitchen, and then you sang instead to feel better. [Tell] What do you think about the steps you accomplished? [Ask]

MARY: I guess I didn't realize I did all that right.

PRACTITIONER: You didn't think you would do as well as you did. [Reflect] One thing to consider is to verbally commit to accepting your feelings instead of avoiding them with eating. You could say it out loud when you practice, and eventually you will automatically say it to yourself. [Tell] What do you think you could say, thinking about what you heard me say when I demonstrated? [Ask]

MARY: It's OK to be angry. I can deal with my mom.

PRACTITIONER: That sounds like a great way to begin to tolerate your distress. [Affirm]

Sustain Talk and Discord

In the context of skills training, sustain talk may sound like desire, ability, reasons, and needs to avoid learning new skills, "I don't really need this. I won't stick to this on my own." Skills training can feel like school, and this may undermine a collaborative stance. Watch out for clients who begin to feel like their skills are poor and their strengths minimal. You need to minimize the expert stance and avoid discord by using the client's own change language about the task (often emerging when eliciting the rationale), maintaining a nonjudgmental stance, and reflecting client concerns. Prevention is the best way to manage sustain talk and discord; however, if counterchange talk is extensive and discord emerges, the strategies discussed in previous chapters are all applicable—for example, emphasizing autonomy, affirming strengths, and shifting focus if necessary.

Planning

Recall that planning encompasses both developing commitment to change and formulating a specific plan of action. Miller and Rollnick (2012) suggest some questions to consider in the planning phase.

"What would be a reasonable next step toward change?"
"What would help this person to move forward?"
"Am I remembering to evoke rather than prescribe a plan?"
"Am I offering needed information or advice with ATA?"
"Am I retaining a sense of quiet curiosity about what will work best for this person?"

Consider transitioning to the planning process by summarizing change talk and the strengths noted in the session so far, followed by a "key question." A key question is an open-ended question that asks what the client's thoughts are about what to do after he or she leaves the session but without pushing for commitment yet. For example, "Mary, we have talked about how you want to figure out how to get people in your life to be more supportive of your weight loss program. This is important to you because you want be able to wear a prom dress in June. Working on problem-solving skills would help you figure this out in different situations, and Sunday lunches at church would be a good place to focus. You practiced the steps and did really well, but exploring all possible solutions before rejecting them is the hardest part, so you realized you need to practice more. So what do you think are your next steps?"

> A key question asks what the client's thoughts are about what to do after the session, but without pushing for commitment.

Although aspects of planning can occur throughout the session, by this point there is typically a clear plan for the next steps such as practicing between sessions and then trying out the skill in the situation of focus. If there is no clear plan, there may be several clear alternatives for reaching the goal. It is then important to guide the client to list the options and to verbalize preferences or "hunches" for the best option to try first. If there are no clear options, then consider brainstorming as described in "Problem-Solving Skills" above before jumping to offering solutions (even in the context of ATA). The next step is to summarize the plan and then discuss the details.

Recall that once the client has chosen a plan for change, you consolidate commitment by (1) developing action steps including implementation intentions (when–then plans); (2) identifying potential barriers to implementation; (3) generating solutions to potential barriers (if–then plans); and (4) reinforcing commitment with open questions to elicit commitment language, scaling questions or rulers, affirming reflections, and expressions of hope and optimism (see Figure 6.2 and Client Handout 6.9).

See how the practitioner promotes the development of if–then plans even when Sam shows evidence of the "false hope syndrome" (see Chapter 4).

PRACTITIONER: Now that we have selected something from your fear hierarchy list, asking someone in a store to help you find something, let's discuss trying to find a time to actually do it.

SAM: Well, my week is pretty full, so I am not exactly sure when I can go to the store.

PRACTITIONER: You are not sure how you will find the time. [Reflect] What ideas do you have in terms of the best days, when you might be near a store? [Open question]

My Plan for Refusal Skills

Changes I would like to make:

Have no more than 1,800 calories a day

Have at least 30 minutes of physical activity a day

These changes are important to me because:

I want to lose 20 lbs. before prom

I want to reach a healthy weight and stay there

I don't want my clothes to be uncomfortable

I want to be able to play sports

I don't want to get diabetes

How refusal skills can help me:

I can reduce pressure and temptations, which will make it easier to stick to

my calorie goal

I can get people to support me without offending them

I plan to take these steps for refusal skills (what, where, when, how):

Avoid my eating triggers whenever possible by:

    1. keeping high-calorie foods out of sight

    2. not going to fast-food restaurants with my friends

    3. asking someone else to get my food at family cookouts and parties

Use the refusal skills from my list when I can't avoid my eating triggers

IF this gets in the way	THEN try this
My family and friends are not supportive despite me talking to them about my goals	Consider spending less time with them for now
Healthier food/drink choices aren't available	Ask what will be available ahead of time and bring my own foods if needed; have smaller portions and drink water
My grandma gets pushy about me having the food she made even when I use my refusal skills	Talk to grandma ahead of time and remind her of what I'm working on, ask mom to be ready to help in advance, or just have a taste and eat later (or eat ahead of time)

FIGURE 6.2. Mary's Change Plan for behavioral and emotion regulation skills.

SAM: Well, on Wednesdays I have a class on the downtown campus, and I suppose I could try to stop in somewhere on my way home.

PRACTITIONER: OK, you came up with a good idea to manage your time. [Affirming reflection] What might get in the way of that? [Open question to identify barriers]

SAM: I think I can do it.

PRACTITIONER: You can't think of anything that might get in the way. [Reflect] Some people say that their schedule changing could be a barrier, what about that? [Open question]

SAM: I guess it is possible that I would need to be somewhere afterward. If it gets to be later, I would need to get home and I don't want to be among all the people on the train, I like earlier trains so that they are less crowded.

PRACTITIONER: So one thing is that if you think it is too late, you would not want to be among the crowds on the train. [Reflect] How might you get around that? [Open question to elicit if–then plan]

SAM: If I make sure I think of it, I can go directly to the store right after class.

PRACTITIONER: You have a great plan [Affirming reflection] How would you remember to do that? [Open question]

SAM: I can write in my class notebook where I take notes to remind myself to go into CVS right after class.

PRACTITIONER: You are committed to getting to the store after school to manage your fear with a small exposure. You came up with a strong if–then plan where you are going to write in your notebook a reminder to go to CVS right after class so you don't have to take a late train. [Summarizing reflection]

The Pregnant Pause

Silence is an important strategy in MI. Filling in silent space is a natural instinct. The pull is especially strong in skills building, when the practitioner is considered an expert teaching a skill that the client does not have. However, allowing for silent spaces gives clients time to cogitate and develop their own (intrinsic) motivation and plans for change. Also, clients differ in how much time they need to process before speaking. Allowing for silences gives clients the space to reflect and then verbalize. Miller and Rollnick (2012) note that a pregnant pause is particularly useful after the summary and key question to increase the likelihood of an intrinsically motivated plan.

> Silence is an important strategy in MI.

MI–CBT Dilemmas

The dilemmas here are quite similar to those when integrating MI with cognitive skills; however, they may be even more challenging because skills involve actively doing something different versus just thinking differently. If the client is not ready to engage in training for a specific skill, and you believe it is a critical skill to address the client's concerns, you have several choices. You can always decide that the particular skill is necessary for the kind of CBT you provide; if clients are not ready to complete the task, they can consider another practitioner. Typically this would occur after multiple attempts to evoke motivation and being honest that the next behavioral step is, in your opinion, the only way to improve the client's difficulties. At this point, the client needs to decide whether he or she is ready to change or would rather take some time to think about changing. You can provide a menu of options for other skills that may address the target concern, being clear that while you believe this is a second choice, the client's preference is your priority. For example, the client may choose to address distress with mindfulness though you believe exposure is more beneficial. Of course, you may ask the client to revisit the skill in the future if progress is not sufficient.

Another dilemma might occur when a client is unwilling to do between-session practice (i.e., homework) or consistently does not do it, and you wonder if skills training is a waste of time without this practice. Choices include reviewing the rationale and utilizing MI strategies to address motivation for between-session practice; engaging the client to practice in the session and prepare for slower progress without between-session practice; or ultimately deciding that CBT cannot work without this practice and refer the client elsewhere. An exploration of the lack of progress (see "Mini-Functional Analysis" above) and helping clients understand the links between limited practice and limited outcomes may increase motivation for between-session practice over time. Again, you and your client may consider a different, or less difficult, skill that the client is ready to practice between sessions. Specifically, using self-monitoring, clients can be encouraged to take smaller steps, to monitor how they feel after taking these smaller steps, and to determine what the outcomes are after the steps. This process will help the client make an informed decision about whether or not to use the skills. See Chapter 7 regarding homework for more detail.

━━━━━━━━━ **ACTIVITY 6.1 FOR PRACTITIONERS** ━━━━━━━━━

Chunk–Check–Chunk

Skills-building sessions typically include the provision of a lot of information. ATA is a foundational skill in MI–CBT integration. Rosengren (2009) suggests the chunk–check–chunk strategy to ensure that you do not overwhelm the client with information and continue to maintain the spirit of MI throughout the interaction, particularly evocation. Provide the information in small chunks, if possible, two to three sentences at a time, and then check with the client for his or her reactions before providing another chunk.

ACTIVITY GOAL: In this activity, you will take skills-related information and break it into chunks as you deliver it to a client, using the chunk–check–chunk strategy. In this way, you will begin to translate CBT into MI–CBT integration.

ACTIVITY INSTRUCTIONS: We provide several examples of skills-related information. Rewrite each section of skills information using the chunk–check–chunk strategy. For each section, write a small chunk of information, write a question to check with the client, and then write the next small chunk of information. Examples of checking questions include: How does that sound? How is this fitting for you so far? How new is this information? How much of this have you heard before? What do you think about this so far? You will create a client response and craft a reflection before the next chunk.

Sample (Not Chunked Information)

Thoughts, feelings, behaviors, and physical responses are connected to each other. What this means is that an emotion can start in any one of those four areas and quickly spread to the other three. As an example of how the four areas fit together, if you are passed over for a promotion at work, you might think, "That's completely unfair. I'm more qualified, and I work harder too! It has to be favoritism." As you have these thoughts, you might have angry feelings. You might do things such as yelling, slamming a door, or sending an angry e-mail. You might have physical responses associated with anger, such as your muscles becoming tense, your heart beat increasing, or your jaw and fists clenching. Believe it or not, you can get control of your emotions by changing the way you respond, starting with just one of the four areas. For most people, the easiest way to do this is to change the way they think.

- *Chunk*: Thoughts, feelings, behaviors, and physical responses are connected to each other. What this means is that an emotion can start in any one of those four areas and quickly spread to the other three.
- *Check*: What do you think about that so far?
- *Client response*: I hadn't really thought about it that way, but it makes sense. Sometimes I hear things that make my head pound and my hands shake. I take that as a signal that the situation is emotionally intense for me.
- *Reflect*: It's a new idea, but it seems to fit together because you've noticed that physical responses can signal a strong emotion for you.
- *Chunk*: As an example of how the four areas fit together, if you are passed over for a promotion at work, you might think: "That's completely unfair. I'm more qualified, and I work harder too! It has to be favoritism." As you have these thoughts, you might have angry feelings. You might do things such as yelling, slamming a door, or sending an angry e-mail. You might have physical responses associated with anger, such as your muscles becoming tense, your heart beat increasing, or your jaw and fists clenching.
- *Check*: How does that fit for you?
- *Client response*: It sounds logical, but it's hard to see how I could recognize all of that happening in the moment.

- *Reflect*: It feels overwhelming, but you see how emotions can affect people in several ways.
- *Chunk*: Believe it or not, you can get control of your emotions by changing the way you respond, starting with just one of the four areas. For most people, the easiest way to do this is to change the way they think.

Your Turn!

First we will depict information that a practitioner might give a client. We will then ask you to try to redo it via chunking, and postulate what a client response might when you elicit feedback. Finally, you will practice reflecting the client's response, trying to reinforce change talk when possible.

Example 1: Information Not Chunked

1. There are several tips that can be helpful to follow when you begin practicing mindfulness. A main goal of mindfulness is to increase your concentration or awareness without responding. Many people find it helpful to pick something to focus on when they get started, such as their breathing, or a simple activity. It's also helpful to practice in a fairly quiet, uncomplicated environment. When you start being mindful, you concentrate on sensations—just noticing things going on around you and inside your body without reacting. If thoughts start to interfere, just let them go without dwelling on them or trying to interpret them. It will get easier to do this with practice. There isn't a set time for how long or how often you practice. The time may vary from a few seconds to several minutes at a time. It may be helpful to give yourself a cue for practicing, such as whenever the phone rings, whenever you sit down or stand up, or while you are brushing your teeth. The choices are yours to make.

Chunk: _____

_____

_____

Check: _____

Client response: _____

Reflect: _____

Chunk: _____

_____

_____

Check: _____

Client response: _____

Reflect: _____

Chunk: _____

_____

_____

Example 2: Information Not Chunked

2. For exposure therapy to be effective, it is important that you experience your anxiety increasing and then decreasing while you are in the anxiety-provoking situation. Leaving the situation while anxiety is high reinforces it. To begin, we make a fear hierarchy, listing your feared situations in order from least to most fearful, rating them on a 10-point scale, with 10 being the most feared situation. For someone with social anxiety, the list might include several different situations such as sitting in a lecture hall with a group of other people, going to see a movie alone, and giving a speech in front of a group of strangers. For the actual exposure activities, we will work together to choose situations from your list. You'll start with one that is in a low to medium position on your list, using the anxiety management skills we've worked on together. You'll gradually work on situations that are higher and higher on your list until your goals have been met.

Chunk: _____

_____

_____

Check: _____

Client response: _____

Reflect: _____

Chunk: _____

_____

_____

Check: _____

Client response: _____

Reflect: _____

Chunk: _____

_____

_____

Example 3: Information Not Chunked

3. It can be difficult to break from your past routines and make different choices. Even well-meaning friends might question why you're not joining in, and that can make it tough to stick with your decision. There are things you can do to make it easier though. If you can plan ahead and avoid situations in which you might be offered a drink, that can take a lot of pressure off of you. For situations that you cannot avoid, you can prepare ahead of time for how you will say "no." We can come up with some responses for you to practice ahead of time that range from a simple "No, thanks," to asking for support by saying something like, "I've been working on drinking less. I know you're being friendly, but I'd really appreciate it if you would stop offering me a beer when I come over. Can I count on you?" Practicing saying these things ahead of time and keeping any explanations short can make it easier for you to say "no" in real situations.

Chunk: _____

_____

_____

Check: _____

Client response: _____

Reflect: _____

Chunk: _____

_____

_____

Check: _____

Client response: _____

Reflect: _____

Chunk: _____

_____

_____

■■■■■ ACTIVITY 6.2 FOR PRACTITIONERS ■■■■■

Sequences: Eliciting and Reinforcing Change Talk for Behavioral and Emotion Regulation Skills

ACTIVITY GOAL: In this activity you will practice developing evoking questions to elicit change talk specifically for skill building. You will then develop a reflection to reinforce the change talk.

ACTIVITY INSTRUCTIONS: For each of the following items, fill in the blanks, making up additional details of the case as necessary in order to practice eliciting change talk for skill building. You will practice completing each of the three components of the sequences. In the first section, you will complete one of the three components of the sequence (question to elicit change talk, client change talk, reflection of change talk). In the second section, you will use your creativity to complete two of the three components.

Item 1

- **Practitioner Strategy to Elicit Change Talk:** What do you hope will happen as a result of working on mood management?

- **Client Change Talk:** I hope I'll stop feeling so irritable. If I can figure out why I snap at people, and why I don't feel like doing anything, then I'm one step closer to being myself again. That's something I've wanted for a long time.

- **Practitioner Reinforcement (Reflection/Question):** _____

_____

Item 2

- **Practitioner Strategy to Elicit Change Talk:** What have you already tried?
- **Client Change Talk:** _____

  _____

- **Practitioner Reinforcement (Reflection/Question):** It's hard to find quiet time, but you have some success when you can get away from the stress of everyday life.

Item 3

- **Practitioner Strategy to Elicit Change Talk:** _____

  _____

- **Client Change Talk:** My family. I can't shake this mood and these worries . . . it's really hurting my marriage. Even my daughter avoids spending time with me. If something doesn't change soon, I think I'm going to lose everyone that matters.
- **Practitioner Reinforcement (Reflection/Question):** You need to make some important changes to bring your family back together.

Item 4

- **Practitioner Strategy to Elicit Change Talk:** Mary, how do you see calorie counting as being helpful to you?
- **Client Change Talk:** _____

  _____

- **Practitioner Reinforcement (Reflection/Question):** _____

  _____

Item 5

- **Practitioner Strategy to Elicit Change Talk:** _____

  _____

- **Client Change Talk:** I'd rather see how to use a phone app. Honestly, I probably wouldn't carry a calorie-counter book around.
- **Practitioner Reinforcement (Reflection/Question):** _____

  _____

Item 6

- **Practitioner Strategy to Elicit Change Talk:** _____

  _____

- **Client Change Talk:** _____

  _____

- **Practitioner Reinforcement (Reflection/Question):** It would always be with you, and it makes the most sense since you're on your phone a lot anyway.

Suggested Responses

Item 1

- **Practitioner Reinforcement (Reflection/Question):** This has been on your mind for a long time, and you want some relief.

Item 2

- **Client Change Talk:** I try to put things out of my mind. It's hard, but if I can have some quiet, then I can relax and it's easier to manage. The trouble is that my life is never quiet. It's busy from one moment to the next.

Item 3

- **Practitioner Strategy to Elicit Change Talk:** What's the most important reason for continuing to work on it?

Item 4

- **Client Change Talk:** I would know when I've had enough—so I don't eat too much.
- **Practitioner Reinforcement (Reflection/Question):** It would help you to stick to your daily goal.

Item 5

- **Practitioner Strategy to Elicit Change Talk:** I can show you how to use a calorie-counter book or a phone app if you'd like.
- **Practitioner Reinforcement (Reflection/Question):** You have a pretty good idea of what would work best for you.

Item 6

- **Practitioner Strategy to Elicit Change Talk:** When could you see yourself using an app?
- **Client Change Talk:** I can use it anytime I eat. I could just look up my foods because I'm on my phone all the time anyway!

Problem Solving

When deciding how to solve a problem, you can create opportunities for success by considering the options and possible outcomes in advance. The problem-solving steps below can be used to identify a problem you want to solve, brainstorm possible solutions, evaluate them, and decide on one to try. Review the example, then fill out your own behavioral experiment form.

SOLVABLE CHALLENGES

Sample:

Problem	• I haven't been able to refill my HIV prescriptions because of my work schedule and I might run out before I can refill them.
Possible solutions	• Call the pharmacy and find out whether I can have them delivered to my aunt's house by mail. • Ask my aunt to pick up my prescriptions for me (she knows my HIV status). • Ask a coworker to cover my shift for a couple of hours (I would have to take a bus to get to/from the pharmacy). • Pick them up on my next day off, which is after I will run out of medication.
Evaluate solutions	• Mailing would be easiest, but I'll still have to go at least a day without medication this month. • My aunt might get mad, but I think she will help unless she has to work (my best option). • Getting my shift covered would give me the time I need, but I don't want my boss to think that I need fewer hours. • I'd have time to get to the pharmacy on my day off, but I'd have to go without medication for a couple of days.
Try one and evaluate	• My aunt picked up my prescription the same day I asked her and said I could ask her anytime. • I talked to my aunt about some of the struggles I've been having with being able to get my medications and get to my clinic appointments. She didn't know that I was having problems and she said that she was really proud of me for trying to take care of myself. I feel like I have a lot more support now. • My aunt asked me if I needed help getting to my clinic appointments.

Before: What do I think is going to happen when I try my solution? *I thought she would help, but that she might be mad that I asked.*

After: What actually happened? *She was happy that I talked to her. She offered to keep helping me.*

My next step will be: *I'm going to ask for help when I need it instead of talking myself out of it.*

(continued)

From *Motivational Interviewing and CBT: Combining Strategies for Maximum Effectiveness* by Sylvie Naar and Steven A. Safren. Copyright © 2017 The Guilford Press. Permission to photocopy this handout is granted to purchasers of this book for personal use or use with clients (see copyright pages for details). Purchasers can download enlarged versions of this material (see the box at the end of the table of contents).

Problem Solving *(page 2 of 2)*

Follow the below skill steps to identify a problem you want to solve, brainstorm possible solutions, evaluate them, and decide on one to try, and then try it and evaluate the outcome.

Problem	
Possible solutions	
Evaluate solutions	
Try one and evaluate	

Before: What do I think is going to happen when I try my solution? _____

_____

After: What actually happened? _____

_____

My next step will be: _____

_____

Behavioral Activation

ACTIVITY SCHEDULING

Part 1: List activities that you enjoy or used to enjoy. Then write how you feel or used to feel when doing the activity and rate the usual strength of that feeling (using the scale at the bottom).

Activities	My Strengths	How I Feel When Doing This Activity	Percent of Feeling
Example: Walking my dog.	I love him and want him to be healthy	Energetic	80
Example: Cooking with daughter	I can cook well and I can help her to be self-sufficient	Happy	75

```
0      10      20      30      40      50      60      70      80      90      100
├───────┼───────┼───────┼───────┼───────┼───────┼───────┼───────┼───────┼───────┤
Feeling not          Mild                Moderate            Strong         Very strong
present                                                                       feeling
```

(continued)

Behavioral Activation *(page 2 of 2)*

Part 2: Keeping Track

Why should you consider making time to do activities that you have enjoyed before?

_____

_____

Keep track of what you do and how your mood changes. List each activity that you do. Then write how you feel when you do it and rate the strength of your feeling.

- How many of your activities are you willing to do each day? _____
- On a scale from 1 to 10, how important is it to you to do them? _____
- Why did you pick that number and not a *lower* number? _____

_____

Date and Time	Activities	Strengths I Used to Get Started	How I Felt When Doing This Activity	Percent of Feeling
4/4/XX 4:00 P.M.	Samples: Walking my dog.	Commitment	Energetic	55
4/4/XX 7:30 P.M.	Cooked dinner with my daughter	Love and pre-planning	Happy	70

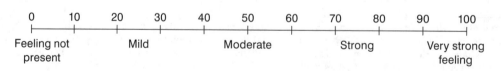

0	10	20	30	40	50	60	70	80	90	100

Feeling not present   Mild   Moderate   Strong   Very strong feeling

Tolerating Distress

Downscaling Emotional Distress

1. My most intense emotion: _____

   _____

2. Strength of my emotion *right now* (or at its most intense point): _____

```
   0     10    20    30    40    50    60    70    80    90   100
   ├──┼──┼──┼──┼──┼──┼──┼──┼──┼──┤
 Feeling not        Mild           Moderate          Strong      Very strong
  present                                                          feeling
```

3. What triggered my emotion: _____

   _____

   _____

   _____

4. My first impulse—what I *want* to do about it: _____

   _____

   _____

   _____

5. Other options that I have:

Things I can change (situation and/or myself)	Ways that I can accept or tolerate the situation

6. The option that I am most willing to consider: _____

   _____

   _____

   _____

(continued)

7. Pros and cons

	Acting on my first impulse	Using my best option instead
Pros		
Cons		

8. Based on my list of pros and cons, what I am going to do is: _____
_____
_____
_____

9. My first step will be: _____
_____
_____
_____

10. This is important to me because: _____
_____
_____
_____

A Simpler Worksheet for Distress Tolerance

The Choice is MINE

I have choices. When I'm feeling _____, then
I can choose how I want to respond.

Emotional Reasons for _____ (Target Behavior)	Alternative Activities
Example: I drink when I feel lonely.	I will watch a movie or go to an exercise class.
Example: I eat when I feel stressed.	I will practice mindfulness.
1.	
2.	
3.	
4.	
5.	
6.	
7.	

Strengths that I can use to help me to do my alternative activities: _____

_____

_____

_____

Three reasons why I think this could work:

1. _____

2. _____

3. _____

Graduated Exposure

Keeping track of how you cope with fearful situations can help you to discover which strategies are the most helpful to you. Start by listing your feared situations, ranging from those that cause very severe anxiety to those that cause mild anxiety. Use this log to track your planned exposure to the situations. For each exposure, rate your level of avoidance, the date you worked on the situation, and the coping strategy you used.

Working through Fear Gradually

	Situation	Fear rating (1–100)	Avoidance (1–100)	Date Exposed	Coping Strategy
1		Highest Rating:			
2					
3					
4					
5					
6					
7					
8					
9					
10		Lowest Rating:			

```
  0      10     20     30     40     50     60     70     80     90    100
  +------+------+------+------+------+------+------+------+------+------+
```

| No anxiety/ avoidance | Mild anxiety/ avoidance | Moderate anxiety/ avoidance | Severe anxiety/ avoidance | Very severe anxiety/ avoidance |

Worry Control

Taming Worry

If I worry less, my life will improve this way: _____

_____

_____

It is important to me to limit my time spent worrying because: _____

_____

_____

To help me to worry less, I will limit worrying to the times below. During these times, I can worry and think about my concerns as much as I want. If I have a worry or concern outside of these times, I will postpone it by using the coping skills that I have been working on, including: _____

_____

_____

START

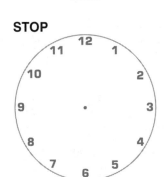

My Thoughts and Concerns

STOP

Refusal Skills

Complete this form to plan how you will respond to social pressure in different situations. Follow the *first step* when possible (avoiding people or situations that trigger you). Identify situations for each refusal skill in the *second step* and use them when needed (communicate your refusal). It is recommended that you practice saying your refusal skills before you use them, which you can do with a counselor, a friend, in front of a mirror, etc. Remember to complete the questions at the bottom of this sheet too!

Refusal Skill	Situations
1. Say "No thank you" assertively.	
2. Give reasons for why you're saying "no."	
3. Suggest alternatives.	
4. Change the subject.	
5. Give reasons for why it will not help with your goal.	

My Refusal Skills goal: _____

Step 1: Avoid the triggers of behavior that will not help you to reach your goal.

Step 2: If it is not possible to avoid triggers, use refusal skills.

My most important reasons for avoiding triggers or using refusal skills are: _____

_____

Some strengths I can use to make choices that will help me to reach my goals: _____

_____

In-Session Skills Training Steps

Write each step of the new skill you would like to learn on the lines below. Then practice the steps with your counselor while following directions at the bottom of the page, starting with WATCH IT.

Learning a New Skill

The Steps

1. _____

2. _____

3. _____

4. _____

5. _____

6. _____

7. _____

WATCH IT: Counselor completes steps and says them at the same time.

How confident are you now to show your counselor? If not very confident, then try WATCH IT AND SAY IT. Otherwise skip to DO IT AND SAY IT.

WATCH IT AND SAY IT: Counselor completes steps and you say the words.

DO IT AND SAY IT: You complete the steps and say the words.

FEEDBACK

What went well: _____

_____

_____

What to focus on during the week: _____

_____

_____

What strengths do I have that will help me: _____

_____

_____

Change Plan for Behavioral and Emotional Regulation Skills

My Plan for _____ **Skills**

Changes I would like to make:

_____

_____

_____

_____

These changes are important to me because:

_____

_____

_____

_____

How _____ skills can help me:

_____

_____

_____

_____

I plan to take these steps for _____ skills (what, where, when, how):

_____

_____

_____

_____

IF this gets in the way   **THEN try this**

_____   _____

_____   _____

_____   _____

_____   _____

_____   _____

CHAPTER 7

Promoting Between-Session Practice and Consistent Session Attendance

We feel it is critical to address how MI might facilitate "homework" in CBT. Why? Homework, or between-session practice, not only is a core element of CBT, but also has been consistently linked to treatment outcomes. In CBT, the explicit focus of the treatment should be how to help clients make changes outside of the therapy sessions, in their real lives. "Homework" is the practice of skills outside of therapy to promote mastery, generalizability to real-world settings, and extension of treatment benefits after termination.

The first meta-analysis of the relationship of between-session practice and treatment success published in 2000 suggested that there existed a small-to-medium effect of homework compliance on treatment outcome across 27 studies, the majority of which were focused on depression and anxiety (Kazantzis, Deane, & Ronan, 2000). The effect was similar for depression and for anxiety and was consistent across the type of homework completed. A follow-up meta-analysis of 23 studies (Mausbach, Moore, Roesch, Cardenas, & Patterson, 2010) found similar effect sizes; again the effect was consistent across the type of homework completed and across target behaviors. However, the authors note that a positive and trusting therapeutic relationship has been significantly related to treatment success regardless of homework (e.g., Green et al., 2008). Thus, if the strategies in this chapter are not successful in increasing homework adherence, engaging skills that demonstrate the spirit of MI will still go a long way in guiding clients to address their concerns.

The First Rule of Homework:
Don't Talk about Homework

For most people, the word "homework" has negative connotations such as "boring," "a chore," and "tedious." Thus, to immediately avoid any counterchange talk

> To avoid any counterchange talk, increase engagement around homework by simply using another term.

or discord, consider increasing engagement around homework by simply using another term such as "practice," "between-session activities," or "take-home exercises." For the rest of this chapter, we will use the term "practice," though some activities (e.g., self-monitoring) are more activity-oriented. The idea is to integrate skills into real-world settings versus practicing them in an unnatural context.

Another preventive step is to convey the spirit of MI (partnership, acceptance, collaboration, and evocation) by carefully discussing the rationale for practice using ATA and reflecting any change talk that emerges regarding practice completion. ATA increases motivation for between-session practice by giving the client the chance to express the rationale for practice and not assuming that clients simply agree with the rationale that you provide. Thus, the first step in addressing lack of homework completion is to make sure that the client agrees with the purposes of the assignments and how they are related to his or her goals. Note that in the example below, the practitioner is able to elicit the rationale with reflections and questions and does not have to provide the rationale with ATA.

PRACTITIONER: Mary, I am wondering why you think it might be important to practice the problem-solving skills we reviewed today between now and the next time we meet? [Ask]

MARY: I'm not sure. I don't have much free time during the week.

PRACTITIONER: You are really not sure why you would want to practice during the week if you are so busy. [Reflect] I am wondering if there are other things you have done that you have had to practice before? [Ask]

MARY: Like you mean band practice? I am supposed to practice my trumpet every night.

PRACTITIONER: You have some experience with practicing skills related to your instrument. [Reflect] What are some reasons why it's important to practice your trumpet? [Ask for change talk]

MARY: So I can get better at it, and I need to learn new songs.

PRACTITIONER: You can see that practice makes you better at it. [Reflect] How would that apply to the problem-solving skills you learned today to help you deal with people who don't support your eating plan? [Ask]

MARY: I guess the more I practice, the better I will be at it.

PRACTITIONER: You realize that practicing makes you better at whatever you want to do, whether it's playing music or improving problem-solving skills. [Reflect] I seem to recall that there were a bunch of things that might be coming up this week that could turn into problems.

MARY: Ugh! I suppose so. There is that whole thing with my sister that I need to figure out.

PRACTITIONER: I just want to make sure that what we agree on for you to do outside of the sessions feels directly related to achieving your goals. [Reflect]

Note that the conversation is eliciting change talk about practicing in general, but you could also evoke change talk around specific assignments—for example: "Why do you think it might be important to record your thoughts during the week?" or "Why would you want to do this behavioral experiment before we meet again?"

Once you have discussed the rationale for between-session practice, consider evoking strategies if you have not heard sufficient change talk and commitment language to move to planning. Recall that you will evoke motivation with open questions to elicit desire, ability, reasons, need, and commitment to change. You can also use strategies such as importance and confidence rulers. Motivation is reinforced when you reflect the responses. Next you elicit a plan for between-session activities so that the client is in the driver's seat in planning the specifics of the plan (see Client Handout 7.1). You have elicited the *why* of the plan with evoking strategies, and now you elicit the other W's: the *what*, the *where*, the *when*, and the *who*.

In terms of the "what" of the plan, provide a menu of options to emphasize personal choice. Be creative so that you can present at least two options. "Mary, for between-session practice, you could use worksheets for possible problems, you could choose some problems that you already know you have to deal with next week and have a list of the steps to deal with them, or maybe you have another idea on how to practice." The next step is to elicit from Mary when she will practice. Forgetting to do between-session practice is often the most common reason why plans for practice fail. Thus, instead of simply determining a day and a time for practice, it is helpful to develop a when–then plan. The "when" is the cue that will prompt Mary to remember to practice—for example, "When I check my e-mail at night, then I will practice." Finally, find out from Mary where she will practice. Once the four W's of the plan have been elicited, discuss potential barriers and make if–then plans to overcome those barriers—for example, "If I lose my worksheets I will have the basic steps of problem solving on my phone." During this discussion, if change talk and commitment language declines (e.g., "I might" instead of "I will"), consider a return to the evoking process or change the plan until there is more solid commitment language.

Missed or Incomplete Assignments

While ambivalence regarding between-session practice is common, significant counterchange talk and discord may not emerge until a client actually returns without having completed what was agreed upon. Missed or incomplete assignments are a sign that motivation has waned even if counterchange talk and discord are not specifically articulated. The excuses for not having done the work outside of the sessions are typically consistent counterchange talk ("I didn't have time"; "I really didn't need it"; "I couldn't manage it this week"). Some common statements include concerns about the time it will take to complete the task, about the task difficulty, about remembering to remember, and about other people finding out about the target concern or treatment. These statements should be addressed using the methods to manage counterchange talk such as reflections and emphasizing autonomy.

> Missed or incomplete assignments are a sign that motivation has waned.

PRACTITIONER: So, how did it go in terms of trying some of the exposures?

SAM: Well, to be honest, I just did not have the time.

PRACTITIONER: It was hard to find the time. [Reflect] What kinds of things got in the way? [Open question]

SAM: I don't know, I just have been real busy in terms of school, classes, and trying to get my homework done, that I just was not able to fit it in.

PRACTITIONER: Yes, you have a lot on your plate. [Reflect] It is really up to you about whether you want to make time for practice, and you said earlier that there were good reasons why practice will help you get better. [Emphasize autonomy]

SAM: Well, my main concern has been on anxiety in talking to others; and the exposures were to try to talk to others and get over it, so I guess it is pretty relevant.

Decisional Balance

Strategies to address counterchange talk and discord are described in Chapter 2 (e.g., reflection without judgment, emphasizing autonomy). However, when change talk is not forthcoming, and counterchange talk predominates, a *decisional balance* activity, as described in dialectical behavior therapy (Linehan, 1993), may help to engage the client in the discussion of ambivalence. Decisional balance was originally conceptualized by Janis and Mann (1977) as a "balance sheet" comparing potential gains (pros) and potential losses (cons), and became a key construct in the "stages-of-change" model where an individual's readiness to change is understood in terms of the balance of pros and cons (Prochaska et al., 1994). The idea is to reduce discord by listening to the cons with reflections, summarizing the cons without judgment, and then asking about potential pros. This can be done as a written or a verbal activity. Miller and Rollnick (2012) emphasize that you rarely want to elicit counter-change talk, but when your strategies to elicit change talk fall flat, this strategy may give you a "running head start" toward a discussion of the pros of change.

Eliciting the Client's View of "Homework Utility"

Yovel and Safren (2007) defined "therapy homework utility" as the strength of the relationship between homework completion and improvement across sessions. Conversely, homework utility could be framed as the relationship between missed homework and no change. We suggest that eliciting or presenting information about this relationship, if strong, can increase client motivation for homework completion. Alternatively, if the relationship is weak and utility is low, then a change in the treatment plan may be warranted. Two strategies from earlier chapters, mini-functional analysis (Chapter 4) and personalized feedback (Chapter 3), can serve to increase motivation by addressing practice utility.

Mini-Functional Analysis

Conduct a mini-functional analysis of antecedents (triggers) and consequences (outcomes) when goals are not met as well as for treatment successes. During this conversation, you may guide the client to consider how between-session practice may contribute to successes and how lack of practice may be hindering goal completion. The idea is to elicit the client's view of this relationship, and if the client spontaneously offers between-session practice as a possible barrier or facilitator to change, you may provide your observations of the utility of practice using ATA. In the example below, Celia has been trying to keep a log of thoughts, feelings, and more helpful thoughts, but her practice has been erratic. Note how the practitioner consistently uses language to support autonomy so that between-session practice is conceptualized as something that the client chose to do versus something prescribed by the practitioner.

> CELIA: Yeah, I can't get out of bed and I get even madder at myself.
>
> PRACTITIONER: It's a vicious cycle. What do you remember about what you wanted to practice to help with these situations? [Open question]

CELIA: I think it was something about thoughts and feelings, but I had such a busy week I forgot.

PRACTITIONER: Right, you wanted to separate the thoughts and feelings on paper and then work on changing the thoughts. [Reflect] It sounds like the week got away from you, and then you had a bad day on Wednesday. [Reflect] What do you see as the relationship between missing practice and having a bad day?

CELIA: I am not sure, but I know that if I don't do something different, things are not going to change.

PRACTITIONER: You can see that if you don't try something different like practicing skills between sessions things might not change like you want them to. [Reflect]

CELIA: Yeah, and something has to change.

PRACTITIONER: You don't want to live like this anymore. What are other times that you didn't try something new, or practice something new that we talked about and things didn't change. [Ask]

CELIA: I'm not sure.

PRACTITIONER: Well, I remember that you had trouble keeping the log and then you felt like the bad situations took over and you couldn't see the good things that happened that week. How do you think that fits with how practice might be related to things not changing for you?

CELIA: I guess if the weeks keep getting away from me, then things will always be like this.

PRACTITIONER: If other things you do during the week take priority over practicing these skills, you will be struggling with these same things more than you want to. [Reflect] What do you think about the time you spend in these struggles versus the time it would take to make a plan to complete these worksheets? [Open question]

You can use a similar approach to discuss the relationship between practice and the client's perceived successes.

PRACTITIONER: You mentioned that you had a really good day on Friday. Tell me about it.

SAM: Well, we had set the goal in here of talking with the person sitting next to me.

PRACTITIONER: You really paid attention to that goal. [Affirming reflection]

SAM: I went down to my seat, and, well, she asked me if I had been in class last time, which I was, and she was not.

PRACTITIONER: You exposed yourself to the situation. [Reflect]

SAM: Yes, I said that I was there, and that I noticed that she was not. Basically we had a conversation. She asked if she could take a look at my notes, and I said she could. I offered to let her take a picture of my notes with her phone, which she did after class, and she thanked me a lot.

PRACTITIONER: So you noticed that when you practiced exposing yourself to a fearful situation, it worked out. You were able to meet your goal of having a conversation, responding to questions, and you even offered extra, to help. [Reflection tying practice to outcome]

SAM: Yeah, I guess so.

PRACTITIONER: And how did it feel beforehand. [Open question]

SAM: Well, leading up to it, I was thinking that I would have to start the conversation, and I was really nervous. I may have shaken a little while waiting for the others to sit down.

PRACTITIONER: So it was hard in the beginning. [Reflect] And then later? [Open question]

SAM: Right afterward, I still felt anxious, but then later in the day and the next day, I felt really good that I actually did this. It has been a long time since I have done that kind of thing.

Personalized Feedback

In Chapter 3, we discussed personalized feedback as a strategy to evoke motivation for change. Personalized feedback involves presenting factual information about target behaviors in an MI style and giving the client space to determine if the information increases his or her concern, desire, reasons, or need for change. What information might be useful to deliver as personalized feedback to increase between-session practice? Yovel and Safren (2007) suggest a *utility index,* calculated by computing the correlation between practitioner ratings of weekly practice completion in the previous week and changes in outcome measurements from the previous week to the current week (e.g., weight, alcohol use, depression symptoms, medication adherence). You can verbally discuss the correlation where higher scores approaching 1 indicate a stronger relationship between utility and change, but it may be more helpful to create a graph demonstrating weekly ratings of practice completion and outcomes (see Figures 7.1 and 7.2).

Utilizing ATA, you will provide only facts, without judgment or immediate analysis of the results, and with statements emphasizing the client's choice and responsibility. You will elicit the client's interpretation of feedback to build motivation for the treatment plan. If utility is high, this should increase client motivation for practice.

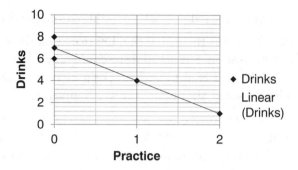

FIGURE 7.1. High homework utility for Carl.

PRACTITIONER: As we decide whether to continue to work on practicing skills or whether to make a change in the treatment plan, would it be OK with you if we look at how practicing has been related to how things are going in terms of alcohol use? [Ask permission]

CARL: That's fine.

PRACTITIONER: More information will help you to make an informed decision. [Reflect and emphasize autonomy] This graph here [Figure 7.1] shows how practice was related to drinking. On this side, practice is rated as 0 for no practice, 1 for partial practice, and 2 for full practice. On this side are the number of drinks you reported for the week. [Tell] What do you think so far?

CARL: So, this graph is for assertiveness skills and whether drinking is related to whether I practiced?

PRACTITIONER: Right. For assertiveness, the line going down shows that in general the more you practiced, the more your drinking went down. [Tell] So what do you think so far? [Ask]

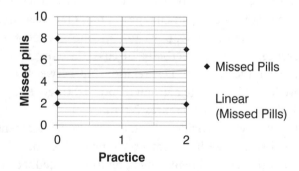

FIGURE 7.2. Low homework utility for Eugene.

CARL: Hmm, it didn't really seem like there was any pattern to my drinking.

PRACTITIONER: It feels like your drinking is up and down, sometimes better and sometimes more than you would like. You see that the graph shows that there might be a pattern with practicing assertiveness skills to less drinking and not practicing the skills to more drinking. [Reflect] What does that pattern mean to you in terms of how you feel about skills practice over the next 2 months? [Open question to elicit change talk]

CARL: I guess I should try to practice more.

PRACTITIONER: You want to focus on assertiveness, and then we can assess again later to see if that's enough or if we need to add other skills. [Reflect]

If utility is low (see Figure 7.2), it may be a sign that practice is ineffective. The reasons for ineffective practice could be related to the quality of the practice or to a mismatch between the assignment and what is necessary for change. Either way, it is a sign that the treatment plan requires collaborative modification.

PRACTITIONER: As we decide whether to continue to work on practicing tolerating distress or whether to make a change in the treatment plan, would it be OK with you if we look at how practicing has been related to how things are going in terms of taking your medications? [Ask permission]

EUGENE: Yeah, is that why we have been doing the pill counts?

PRACTITIONER: The pill counts give you a better assessment on how things are going with your medication so you can decide what you want to do next. [Emphasize autonomy] I have a graph here [Figure 7.2] that shows how practice was related to taking meds each week. On this side, practice is rated as 0 for no practice, 1 for partial practice, and 2 for full practice. On this side are the number of pills you took. [Tell] What do you think so far? [Ask]

EUGENE: Hmmm. Are you sure the practice ratings are correct?

PRACTITIONER: You are wondering how accurate we rated practice. [Reflect] I based this on your report, but of course I could make mistakes. [Tell] If this doesn't make sense, we can redo the graph. Would you like to keep going on this one though? [Ask permission]

EUGENE: Sure. We can decide later if we want to redo it.

PRACTITIONER: OK, you can decide later. [Reflect] Basically the line here and the dots all around suggest that there is not a very strong relationship between practice and taking meds. This could be because we did not get an accurate assessment of practice, because the practice didn't go well, or because distress tolerance is not really helping with taking meds. [Tell with options] What do you think? [Ask]

EUGENE: Hmm, well I like the idea of tolerating distress, but I don't know if that is really why I am missing meds. I am thinking maybe we want to focus on something else and maybe update the graph every week so I can see what's what with the ratings.

PRACTITIONER: You are thinking that maybe we should prioritize other skills. [Reflect] You also want to be more involved in making the graph on a weekly basis. [Emphasize autonomy] Both of those things are great ideas that we can discuss today. [Affirm]

Refer to Chapter 3 for additional tips for delivering feedback.

Session Attendance

The same strategies described above to increase motivation for between-session practice can apply to encouraging session attendance, which can wax and wane throughout treatment. First, an ounce of prevention is worth a pound of cure. Careful attention to eliciting and reinforcing change talk early in treatment can serve to prevent poor treatment retention. Building motivation for addressing the target behavior or symptom, collaborative discussion of the rationale for treatment, and guiding the client to develop his or her own treatment plan, while emphasizing autonomy, all serve to promote session attendance. It is also important to explicitly address the relationship of not completing the between-session work to poor treatment attendance because clients feel bad. The therapist should make it clear that the between-session work is really there to help clients with their problems, and, if they do not do it, it is something that both the therapist and the client need to figure out together. To do this, the client still has to come to the sessions even if he or she did not complete the work that was agreed upon. Of course, it is different when there is a consistent pattern of between-session work not being done. This can open up a discussion about whether or not this is the right time for the client to be in treatment. These strategies can also be done by phone if the client is not attending at all. A discussion of pros and cons can give you an opportunity to express empathy and emphasize personal choice about the cons of attendance while giving you a running start to elicit change talk about session attendance, as in the example below. Note how the counselor briefly elicits cons to express empathy and understanding, thereby paving the way for a more expanded discussion of the pros.

> A discussion of pros and cons can give you an opportunity to express empathy and emphasize personal choice while eliciting change talk.

PRACTITIONER: Hi, Celia. It's great that you agreed to talk by phone so we can see what you want to do next. [Affirm and emphasize autonomy] I am wondering if it would be OK for us to discuss whether continuing treatment makes sense for you. [Ask permission, emphasize autonomy]

CELIA: Yeah, I was scared you might be mad that I haven't showed up. (*Laughs nervously.*)

PRACTITIONER: It can be hard to commit to treatment with all the other things you have going on, and I will support whatever decision you make now and down the road if you decide that is a better time to make a change. [Express empathy, emphasize autonomy]

CELIA: OK, I am just not sure I can do this.

PRACTITIONER: You are torn about whether you can manage to get to appointments. [Reflect] If you would like, we can explore the pros and cons right now and then you can make a decision about what you would like to do. [Ask permission]

CELIA: OK, if we can do it in the next 5 minutes. I have to pick up my daughter.

PRACTITIONER: You have a lot of responsibilities. [Reflect] We can spend the next 5 minutes talking about this and then you can decide if you want to talk further. [Emphasize autonomy] What do you see as some of the disadvantages of continuing treatment? [Ask cons]

CELIA: Mostly time. I am so busy, and it's one more thing to stress me out.

PRACTITIONER: Having so much to do really gets in the way, and you don't want to increase your stress. [Reflect] What are some of the advantages? [Ask pros]

CELIA: Well, if it will help me handle stress, then maybe I can get there!

PRACTITIONER: Treatment could help you manage stress and even though it adds a time commitment, it might be worth it in the long run. [Reflect] What are some other advantages? [Ask pros]

CELIA: My family likes to know that I am doing something to get better.

PRACTITIONER: Your family wants you to work on yourself and you want to show your family that you are doing something to get better. [Reflect]

CELIA: Yes, especially my daughter. But I just don't know.

PRACTITIONER: The main disadvantage is time, and the advantages are that you could handle stress better and show your family that you want to get better. Your daughter is extremely important to you and you want to model for her that you are willing to work on things. [Summary] What do you want to do next? [Key question]

CELIA: Could we make a time to talk by phone next week?

PRACTITIONER: Definitely. We can't do the treatment plan by phone, but we can spend more time discussing a plan to get to sessions if you decide that's what you want to do.

Other options to increase session attendance include returning to the strategies to promote alliance and motivation at the onset of treatment described in Chapter 2 or exploring discrepancies between values and low session attendance using open questions or a values card sort.

MI–CBT Dilemmas

In his seminal report on mental health, the Surgeon General (1999) declared that preventing a problem from occurring is inherently better than having to treat the problem. By using MI skills to demonstrate the MI spirit of partnership, acceptance, compassion, and evocation, you are more likely to prevent noncompliance with treatment tasks and poor session attendance. Although not every session will include every MI process, take time to discuss the rationale for treatment tasks and evoke change talk in every session. If the client is not ready to engage in activities between sessions, you have a choice to make. You may inform the client that practice is necessary for the CBT you provide, and perhaps the client is not ready for CBT at this time. You may decide to see the client for MI-only sessions or have him or her return to see you when he or she is ready to engage in between-session activities. You may decide to provide treatment without assignments but note that progress may be slower. You may then revisit the idea of between-session activities at a later point in treatment. In terms of session attendance, ultimately it is the client's decision whether or not to participate in treatment. You can still convey hope that the client will manage without treatment and emphasize personal choice and responsibility and increase the likelihood that clients will return to you when they are ready for treatment.

ACTIVITY 7.1 FOR PRACTITIONERS

Sequences: Eliciting and Reinforcing Change Talk for Between-Session Practice

ACTIVITY GOAL: In this activity you will practice developing evoking questions to elicit change talk specifically for between-session practice. You will then develop a reflection to reinforce the change talk.

ACTIVITY INSTRUCTIONS: For each of the following items, fill in the blanks and make up additional details of the case as necessary. You will practice completing each of the three components of the sequences. In the first section, you will complete one of the three components of the sequence (question to elicit change talk, client change talk, reflection of change talk). In the second section, you will use your creativity to complete two of the three components.

Item 1

- **Practitioner Strategy to Elicit Change Talk:** How do you think it could be helpful to you to continue exposing yourself to fearful situations this week, such as by starting conversations with people?
- **Client Change Talk:** I can get more comfortable with talking to people that I don't know. It could get easier for me if I do it more.

- **Practitioner Reinforcement (Reflection/Question):** _____

_____

Item 2

- **Practitioner Strategy to Elicit Change Talk:** You have said before that having an easier time talking to people is an important goal of yours.

- **Client Change Talk:** _____

_____

- **Practitioner Reinforcement (Reflection/Question):** Getting past your fear of talking to people is an important step toward reaching your other goals—like having friends to go out with.

Item 3

- **Practitioner Strategy to Elicit Change Talk:** _____

_____

- **Client Change Talk:** Good question. I think I'd have to start at least two or three more conversations before I try the next step.
- **Practitioner Reinforcement (Reflection/Question):** You are getting close, but you need a little more practice first.

Item 4

- **Practitioner Strategy to Elicit Change Talk:** Carl, you mentioned a few minutes ago that you didn't have a chance to practice your refusal skills again this week because you didn't have time. I'm wondering if we can talk about that and come up with a solution that would be helpful to you.

- **Client Change Talk:** _____

_____

- **Practitioner Reinforcement (Reflection/Question):** _____

_____

Item 5

- **Practitioner Strategy to Elicit Change Talk:** _____

  _____

  _____

  _____

- **Client Change Talk:** Well . . . since you brought it up, yeah, I guess I do feel that way. It's not that I think that I can't do it, because I can. I'm just not sure it would work, like you said. Honestly, I know my family and they are just going to push me harder if I say no. I don't see it working with them and it would put me in an awkward position.

- **Practitioner Reinforcement (Reflection/Question):** _____

  _____

  _____

  _____

Item 6

- **Practitioner Strategy to Elicit Change Talk:** _____

  _____

- **Client Change Talk:** _____

  _____

- **Practitioner Reinforcement (Reflection/Question):** You'd like to test out your skills with others before you use them with family.

Suggested Responses

Item 1

- **Practitioner Reinforcement (Reflection/Question):** Practicing more could really build your confidence.

Item 2

- **Client Change Talk:** It is. I feel like I could start doing other things, like making friends and going out to have fun, if I can get over this fear of talking to people.

Item 3

- **Practitioner Strategy to Elicit Change Talk:** How much practice starting conversations do you think you need before you are ready to try the next step on your list?

Item 4

- **Client Change Talk:** The end of the week just seemed to sneak up on me. I was planning to practice, but it never happened.
- **Practitioner Reinforcement (Reflection/Question):** You wanted to try out the skills we worked on even though life was moving pretty fast.

Item 5

- **Practitioner Strategy to Elicit Change Talk:** Sometimes, when people have trouble finding time to practice, what they are telling me is that they are not sure that the skill will be helpful to them—or that they are not sure they can do it—even when part of them wants to do the practice. I'm wondering if you're having thoughts like that too.
- **Practitioner Reinforcement (Reflection/Question):** That's really helpful to hear. I'm glad you can talk to me about it. The practice ideas that we come up with are meant to be helpful to you, but I can see that you're frustrated. You know your situation best, and the steps you take are your choice.

Item 6

- **Practitioner Strategy to Elicit Change Talk:** We could talk about other options for practicing your refusal skills, or whether this is the right time in treatment for you to use refusal skills. Or maybe you have other thoughts.
- **Client Change Talk:** Let's talk about some other options. I guess I have to see how it works before I do it with my family.

▰▰▰▰▰▰▰ ACTIVITY 7.2 FOR PRACTITIONERS (AND FOR CLIENTS!) ▰▰▰▰▰▰▰

The Experience of Building Motivation for Practice

Skills practice is an important ingredient for successful CBT, but it isn't easy! Consider how you have been practicing the skills discussed in these chapters. Have you completed the activities at the end of the chapters so far? Your reasons for limited practice are likely similar to those of your clients. See if the strategies we suggest for clients work to shift your motivation. *Consider using the same activities for your clients as a client handout.*

ACTIVITY GOAL: In this activity you explore your own motivation for MI–CBT skills practice using strategies described in this chapter.

ACTIVITY INSTRUCTIONS: Choose a practice goal such as completing the activities or in this book, practicing MI–CBT in general, or a specific MI–CBT skill (e.g., ATA, discussing rationale, setting agenda, reflections), and then complete the exercises for the behavior.

Practice Behavior: _____

Exercise 1. Importance Ruler: Mark on the ruler how important you feel this practice behavior is to change.

```
    1     2     3     4     5     6     7     8     9    10
    ├──┼──┼──┼──┼──┼──┼──┼──┼──┼──┤
  Not at all important      Somewhat important      Extremely important
```

Why did you choose this number and not a lower number? _____

_____

_____

Exercise 2. Pros and Cons: List the pros and cons of _____ (the practice behavior). Circle the biggest PRO.

<u>Cons of Practicing</u>   <u>Pros of Practicing</u>

_____   _____

_____   _____

_____   _____

_____   _____

Exercise 3. Values–Behavior Discrepancy: Review this list of values and circle your top three values and then answer the questions that follow the values list.

Attractive
(Looking good inside or out)

Independent
(Being in control of myself)

Spiritual
(Having spiritual or religious beliefs)

Healthy
(Having good health)

Honest
(Being truthful)

Hopeful
(Being positive or full of hope)

Loved
(Being loved or giving love to others)

Happy
(Feeling glad or having a happy mood)

Responsible
(Being someone
others can trust or count on)

Organized
(Being neat or having things in order)

Dedicated
(Sticking with something)

Successful
(Moving toward my goals
or reaching my goals)

Role Model
(Being someone others look up to)

Good Communicator
(Being heard or understood by others)

Athletic/Fit
(Being physically active)

Good Cook
(Being able to make foods
that taste good or people enjoy)

Relationships
(Having strong family, friend,
or romantic relationships)

Confident
(Being sure of myself
or feeling like I can reach my goals)

Self-Respect
(Caring about or taking care of myself)

Accepted
(Being respected or included by others)

Now respond to the following questions:

If you decide not to practice, how will it interfere with these values? _____

_____

_____

_____

If you decide to practice more, how will it help you live out these values? _____

_____

_____

_____

The Five W's for Between-Session Practice

Complete the activity below to plan your skill practice. Doing so will help you to determine the five W's: *what* you will do, *where* and *when* you will do it, *why* it is important and why you feel confident that you can do it, and *who* will help you if needed.

My Practice Planner

1. My planned practice activity: _____

   _____

   _____

   _____

   _____

2. When and where I plan to do my practice: _____

   _____

   _____

   _____

3. *Importance* of doing my practice as planned:

0	10	20	30	40	50	60	70	80	90	100

   Not at all   Mild   Moderate   Strong   Very
   important   important

   Why did you pick that number and not a lower number? _____

   _____

   _____

4. My *confidence* that I can do my practice as planned:

0	10	20	30	40	50	60	70	80	90	100

   Not at all   Mild   Moderate   Strong   Very
   confident   confident

   Why did you pick that number and not a lower number? _____

   _____

   _____

(continued)

5. Possible barriers and how I'll handle them:

Things that could stop me from practicing	Things I can do to make sure that I practice anyway/who can help

CHAPTER 8

Maintenance

Once someone has achieved his or her goals for change, the maintenance of change can be difficult across a broad spectrum of concerns associated with mental and physical health. Following initial treatment, more than half of all individuals do not maintain behavior changes. This is true in many domains, including substance use, physical activity, nutrition, depression, and other long-term mental health conditions (Keller & McGowan, 2001; McKay et al., 1999; Miller & Hester, 1986; Piasecki, 2006; Wing & Phelan, 2005). Because MI was originally developed to build motivation for *initial* change, MI strategies for *maintaining* change have been less specified. But many clients need additional support for maintenance beyond the change. Motivation continues to fluctuate after clients have enacted changes, and the integration of MI and CBT during the process of maintaining change may bolster CBT approaches to "relapse prevention" (e.g., Beck, 2011; Marlatt & Donovan, 2005).

In specifying cognitive therapy approaches, Beck (2011) suggests that there are certain strategies you can use *throughout* treatment to increase the likelihood of maintenance. These strategies are consistent with the practitioner skills described in earlier chapters including reflections of progress, functional analysis of positive behavior change, and affirming statements. Originally focusing on substance use, Marlatt and Donovan (2005) describe specific strategies to implement *after* successful treatment to prevent relapse including an assessment of triggers, review and practice of coping skills to manage those triggers, preparing for setbacks with coping skills, and normalizing lapses. Beck (2011) and Marlatt and Donovan (2005) both suggest tapering sessions and considering booster sessions after termination, and both note the importance of self-efficacy and social support. In this chapter, we address the integration of MI with those CBT strategies that address maintenance of change after the initial treatment plan has resulted in a positive outcome.

Engaging

The first tenet of engaging is to avoid the term "relapse." Miller argues that using the term "relapse" assumes that there are only two states regarding maintaining change: success or failure (Miller, Forcehimes, & Zweben, 2011). The true course of maintenance of behavioral change is a process of ebbs and flows, with returns to an ambivalent, preintervention behavior being highly variable in frequency and intensity. Thus, MI–CBT integration suggests avoiding the terms "lapse" and "relapse." Instead, express empathy to your client about the difficulties of maintaining changes in the context of temporary setbacks or slips, elicit the client's perspective on temporary slips, and support autonomy and choice in returning to the path of change.

The "goal violation effect" refers to the phenomenon of giving up the pursuit of behavior change in the face of a setback. It was initially presented in Marlatt's model of relapse prevention for addiction, and referred to as the "abstinence violation effect" (Marlatt & George, 1984). If clients view setbacks or slips as irreparable failures, they find it much harder to return to maintenance. Taking the position that slips should be viewed as learning experiences can help maximize the chances of longer-term maintenance. Thus, expressing empathy about slips is an important part of engaging. Consider a "normalizing reflection," a reflection that adds a word or statement indicating that what the client is expressing is a normal part of the change process. Discussing the difference between a "slip" and a "relapse" using ATA can help prevent the violation effect.

> Viewing slips as learning experiences improves the chances of long-term maintenance.

> PRACTITIONER: If it's OK with you, it might be helpful to discuss the differences between what people call a relapse and what is normal when you are maintaining all the changes you have made. [Ask]
>
> EUGENE: Sure. I know a relapse is like when you mess up.
>
> PRACTITIONER: If you forget to take medications, it's like messing up. [Reflect] Making mistakes like forgetting your medication sometimes is normal. Nobody is perfect, but it doesn't mean you are back to square one like when you first started. [Tell]

EUGENE: I'm scared of getting sick again or infecting my boyfriend if my viral load goes up.

PRACTITIONER: It makes sense that you would feel scared to lose the changes you have made. [Reflect] Being gentle with yourself when you have slips and then getting back on track is part of the process and might work better than beating yourself up and falling back into old patterns. What do you think of that approach, thinking about slips instead of a full relapse? [Ask]

EUGENE: My mom always said everybody makes mistakes, so I need to be OK with that.

After the client has initial success making changes, it is not uncommon for him or her to consider whether treatment is still necessary. In the context of expected temporary setbacks, it may be necessary to renew motivation for the treatment plan to support the maintenance of change. Spend time discussing the rationale in advance with ATA. Offer a normalizing reflection, emphasizing that ambivalence about continuing treatment to maintain changes is not unusual. You can further support autonomy by offering choice about the maintenance phase of treatment (e.g., frequency of sessions, boosters), as in the following example.

PRACTITIONER: Why do you think it might be important to identify what leads to a slip into overeating? [Ask]

MARY: Well, I guess that way I can avoid these things.

PRACTITIONER: We can spend the next few sessions figuring out how to cope with these triggers. That might help you maintain the changes you have made in your eating. [Action reflection and tell] What do you think of starting a list of triggers today? [Ask]

MARY: That would be fine. How long will it take?

PRACTITIONER: You are wondering when you will be done with treatment. [Reflect] That would be up to you. [Support autonomy] We could take the next few sessions to practice skills to manage triggers and talk though any slips, which are common when you are working on maintaining changes. [Tell] What do you think of that approach? [Ask]

MARY: OK. I still get tempted all the time.

PRACTITIONER: You still feel that normal temptation to overeat. [Normalizing reflection] Although we were wrapping up, we can continue to meet weekly until you feel stronger about overcoming the temptation, or we can switch to every other week and then down to once a month when you feel ready. [Provide menu of options]

Focusing

After initial treatment plan objectives are collaboratively considered complete, maintenance sessions often begin with a process of refocusing. Recall that focusing is the collaborative process of determining the scope of the conversation, which can include goals and tasks as well as thoughts, feelings, and concerns. In the maintenance phase of treatment, values and goals may have changed, and exploration of the client's current concerns can help to refocus treatment on goals for maintenance of change that are consistent with current values.

> PRACTITIONER: Now that we have moved through basically all of the items on your hierarchy for anxiety, what do you think is next? [Open question]
>
> SAM: Well, I am not quite sure, Doc, but I do think that things were difficult at first, but now if I really push myself, I can do what I need to do.
>
> PRACTITIONER: You sure have made a lot of progress. [Reflect] How does that feel? [Open question]
>
> SAM: It feels good, but I also really don't want to get back to where I was.
>
> PRACTITIONER: You want to keep at it so you don't go back to how things were. [Reflect] We can discuss what might be the next steps to maintain these changes.
>
> SAM: Yes, I was wondering about that.
>
> PRACTITIONER: So we had started considering three separate goals, the first was working on your anxiety, the second your depressed mood due to lack of enough friendships, and the third on drinking. [Summarizing reflection]
>
> SAM: Yes, so now I think I have my anxiety under control, but I still do not really have new friends.
>
> PRACTITIONER: So you still have some goals around making friends. [Reflect] And what about your mood? [Open question]
>
> SAM: That is a bit better, but I do still wish I had some friends at school.
>
> PRACTITIONER: So your mood is a little better, but making friends at school is your main goal now. [Reflect]
>
> SAM: That might be harder than the exposures but maybe not.
>
> PRACTITIONER: Even though the exposures were hard, you made it through them. [Affirming reflection] So now you would like to focus on making friends, maybe using the same step-by-step approach. [Action reflection]

A collaborative assessment of potential triggers and possible coping plans can serve to focus on specific objectives for the maintenance phase of treatment (see

Client Handout 8.1). For clients who are not able to easily identify triggers, a guided interview or functional analysis is recommended by many CBT approaches (e.g., Witkiewitz & Marlatt, 2007). The antecedents may be intrapersonal (emotions, thoughts) or interpersonal (people, places, situations), and these triggers are likely linked according to the cognitive model. In the maintenance phase it is especially important to determine not only the triggers for slips but also the antecedents and consequences for successful behavior change. This information will support coping plans to manage triggers.

As previously described in Chapter 3, you integrate MI into the assessment process by balancing reflections and questions and pausing to summarize and "connect the dots." Use action reflections to embed potential coping strategies into reflections. Recall that there are three subtypes of action reflections: behavioral suggestion, cognitive suggestion, and behavior exclusion. The following examples demonstrate how to incorporate action reflections to move from the *why* to maintain to the *how* to maintain.

Action Reflection with Behavioral Suggestion: When you feel alone, that's when you are more likely to eat, and identifying the right people to support you might help you avoid this trigger.

Action Reflection with Cognitive Suggestion: When you feel alone, that's when you are more likely to feel depressed, and figuring out how to tolerate those alone feelings might help you manage this trigger.

Action Reflection with Behavior Exclusion: When you feel alone, you try to talk to your boyfriend but that doesn't always work because you're not sure you can rely on him, so thinking of some other strategies might be helpful.

TIP for Focusing: Tolerate Uncertainty

In Chapter 1, we described the righting reflex, the human tendency to correct things that are perceived as wrong. This reflex often translates into premature problem solving and advice giving, both counter to the MI spirit. For several reasons, the righting reflex may be particularly strong in the maintenance phase of treatment. First, you might feel that the alliance is strong and so believe that the client may tolerate more advice giving and problem solving. Second, because you now know the client very well compared to at the onset of treatment, you may feel pulled to provide information or advice based on this knowledge, rationalizing to yourself that you are still being client-centered because it is based on what you know about the client. Third, when your client is first beginning to improve, you may feel increased pressure to take responsibility for treatment in his or her fragile state instead of giving the client space to learn from potential slips. Finally, you may feel rushed as termination is near, pulling you to provide information or advice as a way of moving the maintenance phase along.

However, as noted above, engagement is still a critical process in the maintenance phase when motivation may wax and wane. Providing solutions for your clients may undermine their ability to serve as their own guides. Increasing your tolerance for uncertainty will allow you to resist the righting reflex. Tolerating ambiguity in the identification of triggers and associated coping plans allows them to emerge through the interview process as well as through exploring slips as they occur. In this way, you ensure that the client is still in the driver's seat when focusing in the maintenance phase while you continue to help navigate in the passenger seat.

Evoking

You may feel pulled to rush the evoking process in the maintenance phase. However, high rates of setbacks across behaviors and conditions underscore the importance of this process. Renewing commitment after slips is particularly important to prevent further slips. We address specific ways to evoke motivation for maintaining changes, including specificity of language to evoke motivation for maintenance, understanding the role of outcome expectancies, exploring discrepancies between values and goals, and supporting self-efficacy.

Specificity of Language

MI is goal-oriented, and in MI–CBT integration you are guiding the client toward a clear change objective. Motivation can waiver based on the specificity of this goal. For example, a client may express relatively high motivation to continue the progress he or she has made, but upon your further inquiry may reveal him- or herself to be more ambivalent about maintaining a behavior in the context of certain triggers. Thus, you must use language that elicits and reinforces change talk and commitment about the specific maintenance objective determined in the focusing process.

The specificity of your language is important here. Whereas change talk in earlier phases of treatment may address change in general, change talk about maintenance is specific about maintaining changes (e.g., "It is important for me to *stay* sober because I don't want to go back to being unemployed"; "I like the way I am feeling since I lost weight and I want it to *stay* that way"). Change talk about maintenance may also include desires, ability, reasons, needs, and commitment to maintaining change (e.g., "I know I need to keep coming to sessions even though I am feeling better because I don't want to start all over again"). Thus, use your strategies to elicit change talk about maintenance and then reinforce it (e.g., with reflections). In the following example, see how the practitioner specifically elicits and reinforces change talk about maintenance with open questions and reflections specific to maintaining changes.

> PRACTITIONER: Celia, you have made some very difficult changes. Why do you feel that you need to maintain these changes? [Ask]
>
> CELIA: Well, at first I was really doing this for my family, but now I am doing this for myself. I like who I am now a lot better than before.
>
> PRACTITIONER: You want to maintain these changes because you like who you are now and you want to stay that way. [Reflect]

Similarly, your evoking strategies (see Chapters 4 and 7), such as an importance ruler, will also be specific for maintenance.

> PRACTITIONER: Carl, on a scale of 1 to 10, how important is it for you to maintain sobriety now that probation is over? [Evoking question]
>
> CARL: Probably about a 6.
>
> PRACTITIONER: Somewhere in the middle, but toward more important. [Reflect] Why did you say a 6 and not a lower number for maintaining the changes you have made? [Open question to elicit change talk]
>
> CARL: I thought I would start drinking as soon as I didn't have to pee in a cup, but my family is so much happier now.

> Change talk in earlier phases of treatment addresses change in general; change talk in this phase focuses on *maintaining* changes.

> PRACTITIONER: It is important for you to maintain the changes you made because you want your family to stay happy and not go back to how things were before. [Reflect change talk]

Outcome Expectancies

The client's thoughts following a slip are considered a key determinant of whether the person is likely to slip further (Marlatt & Donovan, 2005). Individuals who have positive outcome expectancies around engaging in the target behavior (e.g., Drinking will help me relax) or negative outcome expectancies about maintaining change (If I go to this party, I will get anxious) are more likely to have difficulty maintaining changes. Exploring desire, ability, reasons, and needs for maintaining changes supports outcome expectancies in favor of change. Although you can elicit reasons to avoid old negative behaviors (avoidance goal), there is some evidence to suggest that emphasizing change talk and commitment language about *maintaining* new behaviors (maintenance goal) may be even more important (Nickoletti & Taussig, 2006; O'Connell, Cook, Gerkovich, Potocky, & Swan, 1990). For example, when discussing slips, it may be fruitful to elicit change talk about the enjoyment of exercise and returning to the gym, the feeling of relaxation when using mindful meditation, or the positive mood experienced when scheduling pleasurable activities, instead of avoiding video games or lying in bed during the day. This may increase the likelihood of reengagement and continued participation into a more habitual activity.

Developing Discrepancy

Another way to elicit change talk about maintenance is to explore discrepancies between the person's values and goals and slips or setbacks. First, reflect values already discussed and explore new values and goals developed since the client experienced initial behavior change. Then, express empathy around short-term needs (e.g., managing stress), which may be in conflict with long-term values and goals (e.g., preventing chronic physical illness), especially after a slip. A double-sided reflection can be used to highlight the discrepancy with empathy: *"It must be hard to avoid overeating when you are stressed, yet you say it's important to you not to have to have to worry about diabetes."* Highlighting discrepancy can be followed by an evocative open question: *"What do you want to do, if anything, to get back on track?"*

Increasing Self-Efficacy

As noted above, self-efficacy is considered to be a key predictor of maintenance success (Beshai, Dobson, Bockting, & Quigley, 2011; Herz et al., 2000; Lam & Wong, 2005; Marlatt & Donovan, 2005; Minami et al., 2008; Nigg, Borrelli, Maddock, & Dishman, 2008); however, few maintenance interventions specify exactly how to support self-efficacy. The skills-building steps, as described in the previous chapter, are ways to increase feelings of competence. Continue to use these steps (modeling, rehearsal, and feedback) to practice coping skills to manage triggers.

Additional strategies to support efficacy after slips may be necessary. Continue to use affirmations ("You are very persistent in your goals") and open questions to elicit change talk about the ability to maintain change ("How have you maintained changes in the past?"). Elicit strengths that the client has used to achieve difficult changes to date ("What strengths did you use that helped you get your viral load down?"). When a client does not easily identify personal strengths, particularly in relation to maintenance, an exploration of what others (friends, family) say about the client's strengths may be fruitful ("You mentioned that your mom says you are a very strong person. How might being a strong person help you maintain the changes you have made in your drinking?"). Another strategy is to directly convey hope and optimism regarding the client's ability to maintain changes. This does not have to be a blanket belief in change, but can be linked to certain constraints.

For example, "I believe you can get back on track [after a slip] when you get the help you need from your family." Research suggests that practitioner optimism is a common factor evident in positive therapeutic outcomes (Lambert & Barley, 2001).

Polivy and Herman (2002) emphasize an important point about self-efficacy. They define the "false hope syndrome" as "unrealistic expectations about the likely speed, amount, ease, and consequences of self-change attempts" (p. 677). Overconfidence and setting unrealistic goals often undermines successful change. In fact, their review suggests that having enough self-efficacy that is realistic (i.e., that is earned by the client's experience) at the end of treatment is more predictive of success than self-efficacy at the onset of treatment when it has not yet been "earned." Thus, tying confidence to specific successful change attempts from the past and successful learning of skills will be more powerful than generic expressions of hope and optimism. This false hope syndrome also has implications for planning, as described below.

Planning

Individuals who set rigid "all or nothing" goals are more likely to view slips as failure and experience the goal violation effect. When goals are flexible, an individual is more likely to return to positive behavior change after a slip (e.g., Marcus et al., 2000; Marlatt & Gordon, 1985). For example, from the traditional Alcoholics Anonymous (AA) perspective, clients can think about planning for "one day at a time" instead of viewing a rigid goal of permanent abstinence (or, in the case of depression, say, never feeling depressed again). That is not to say that abstinence cannot be the client's ultimate goal, but a flexible short-term goal can allow for the normalization of slips or setbacks. Hence, offering a menu of options can support flexible goal setting while also supporting autonomy and therefore maximizing the chances of maintenance. Additionally, by offering a menu, there is less likelihood

> A flexible short-term goal can allow for the normalization of slips or setbacks.

of a client rejecting a suggestion, while you support the idea that there are multiple paths to success. If one is not successful, another may be considered in the future.

Specifying a maintenance change plan is similar to the components of making plans for initial change (e.g., summarize change talk, develop short-term steps, elicit potential barriers, and discuss if–then plans), but the language is about maintenance. This includes summarizing change talk about maintaining changes, eliciting short-term steps for coping skills development, discussing potential barriers, developing if–then plans for avoiding triggers, and determining between-session practice to enact coping plans to support maintenance (see Client Handout 8.2 and Figure 8.1 for a sample). Consider including booster sessions as part of if–then

---

My Plan

Changes I would like to maintain:

Stay sober

Keep sadness rating above 20 on 0–100 scale

Continue working on improving my relationship with my wife

Maintaining these changes are important to me because:

I need to stay out of legal trouble and prison

I want to keep my wife to be happy

I want to show everyone that I can stay sober

I am looking forward to waking up every day now and I want that feeling to continue

I plan to keep doing these things to maintain my changes (what, where, when, how):

Keep doing activity scheduling and do the activities every single day

Keep using my refusal skills and managing my cravings

Continue using anger management

Keep working on my communication skills and read the "tips" handout at least once
a week

IF this gets in the way	THEN try this
I lose motivation after an argument with my wife	Remind myself of my successes and why it is important to me to keep trying
	Return to therapy if I have trouble maintaining motivation (if I start telling myself to "forget it" or "it's not worth it")
I get too busy to do my scheduled activities	Reprioritize my schedule to keep doing at least one activity a day and remind myself of how doing them has helped me
I have a sobriety slip	Use my SLIP plan
	Return to therapy if I have more than one slip in a month

FIGURE 8.1. Carl's Change Plan for maintenance.

plans. If during the maintenance planning process, clients are unable to detail how they will accomplish their goals and overcome potential barriers, this may be a sign of having false hope. You may then need to guide them toward a more realistic goal and plan.

Social support has long been identified as a predictor of maintenance (e.g., Havassy, Hall, & Wasserman, 1991; Perri, Sears, & Clark, 1993). There are several methods used to increase social support to maintain behavior change. Interventions across multiple behavioral domains often include a spouse or other family member (Anderson, Wojcik, Winett, & Williams, 2006; Bird et al., 2010; Kiernan et al., 2012; Lobban & Barrowclough, 2009; Orsega-Smith, Payne, Mowen, Ho, & Godbey, 2007; Westmaas, Bontemps-Jones, & Bauer, 2010). Encouraging participation in support groups is another method (Amati et al., 2007; Douaihy et al., 2007). Individual-level interventions may have skills training components specifically addressing the identification of social support, communicating with supportive others, and the avoidance of negative social influences (Marlatt & Donovan, 2005; Westmaas et al., 2010). Finally, you may offer a menu of options for if–then plans to overcome barriers that include social support (e.g.,"If I don't feel like going for a walk, I will call a friend to join me").

TIP for Final Planning: The Termination Session

The following are essential elements of a termination session (see Figure 8.2). First, ask the client for his or her own perceptions of positive changes and reflect and affirm them. Second, tell your own perceptions of positive changes in an affirmation, making sure to attribute changes to the client's thoughts, feelings, and behaviors and not your own efforts. These statements should be positive and relatively free of qualifiers like, "Even though you . . ." or "Except for. . . ."

Third, explore termination feelings with open questions and use normalizing reflections. Fourth, express hope and optimism for the future, tailoring

- Ask about the client's perception of positive changes throughout treatment.
- Reflect and affirm.
- Tell your own perception of positive changes in an affirmation.
- Explore termination feelings with open questions and reflections.
- Express specific hope and optimism based on client strengths.
- Give menu of options for future contact.
- Develop an ongoing change plan.
- Highlight the journey with a summary that includes where the client started, where he or she has ended, affirmations, and specific examples of change talk the client gave along the way.

FIGURE 8.2. Checklist of essential elements for a termination session.

your statements based on your knowledge of the client ("Given the persistence you have had with all these challenges, I believe you will continue to work toward your goals"). Fifth, give a menu of options for phone contact, booster sessions, or continued treatment. Finally, finish with the best possible summary, incorporating where the client started, where he or she has finished, and embed the best examples of the client's change talk and commitment language.

MI–CBT Dilemmas

A key dilemma is when to move on to the maintenance phase. In MI–CBT, you do not choose—rather, it is a collaborative decision. If you have followed this guide so far, you and your client have collaboratively developed a treatment plan with specific objectives and have modified this plan throughout treatment. Do you prepare for termination when objectives have been met? When symptoms have completely remitted? When abstinence has been achieved for a period of time? When the client is no longer engaged in the target behavior? What happens if the client wants to prepare for termination, but you think further treatment is necessary? What happens when you believe the client is ready for maintenance and termination but the client does not? We delineate these dilemmas, but we cannot provide answers as the decision is between you and your client. Using ATA, you elicit clients' perceptions, provide your own perspective, and then elicit their response.

We believe, ultimately, that it is the client's decision. You and your client may disagree about whether treatment is close to termination, but completion of treatment objectives to the client's satisfaction may be a good indicator that it is time to move into the maintenance phase. Similar to discussion of dilemmas in previous chapters, if you believe the client is not ready, you can be honest about your opinion using ATA. You can still convey hope that the client's preference for termination will work, building the alliance so that your advice can be considered in the future if the client is still struggling.

━━━━━━━━━━━━━ **ACTIVITY 8.1 FOR PRACTICIONERS** ━━━━━━━━━━━━━

Eliciting and Reinforcing Change Talk about Maintenance

Change talk in the earlier phases of treatment may address desire, ability, reasons, need, and commitment toward making initial changes or behavior change in general. Change talk about maintenance is specifically about maintaining changes—for example: "It is important for me to *stay* healthy because I like having energy"; "I like the way I am feeling since I started exercising and I want it to *stay* that way." Change talk about maintenance may also include desire, ability, reasons, needs, and commitment to the maintenance phase of treatment—for example: "I know I need a few more sessions because I want to make sure I don't slip back."

To elicit change talk about maintenance, the language you use must be specific to maintenance, both in terms of the strategies to elicit change talk and the skills to reinforce change talk.

ACTIVITY GOAL: In this activity you will practice how to elicit and reinforce change talk about maintenance.

ACTIVITY INSTRUCTIONS: Each statement below is designed to elicit change talk or to reinforce change talk with reflections or open questions. Edit the statement to elicit and reinforce change talk about maintenance. Some words to consider are "maintain," "continue," "stay," "keep up," "keep it going," "remain," "preserve," and "persist."

Examples

1. What are some of the reasons why you want to stop drinking?
   Open questions to elicit change talk: What are some of the reasons why you want *to continue* to cut back on your drinking?
2. So you would like to exercise to have more energy.
   Reflection to reinforce change talk: So you would like *to continue* to exercise to have more energy.

Your Turn!

1. What kinds of things would be better if you ate more fruits and vegetables?

   Open questions to elicit change talk: _____

   _____

   _____

2. You want to get along better with your daughter.

   Reflection of change talk: _____

   _____

   _____

3. You think taking medication will keep you going for your family.

   Reflection of change talk: _____

   _____

   _____

4. On a scale of 1 to 10, how confident are you that you can practice mindfulness?

   Open questions to elicit change talk: _____

   _____

   _____

5. What would be the best thing that would happen if you managed to lose some weight?

    Open questions to elicit change talk: _____

    _____

    _____

6. What is the worst thing that would happen if you don't schedule these activities?

    Open questions to elicit change talk: _____

    _____

    _____

7. You feel like you are more in control when you take your medications.

    Reflection of change talk: _____

    _____

    _____

8. Why is it important to you to practice pushing through your anxiety in social situations?

    Open questions to elicit change talk: _____

    _____

    _____

9. You value your family. How does working on your depression fit with that value?

    Open questions to elicit change talk: _____

    _____

    _____

Managing Slips

Everyone has a slip from time to time. You can stop a slip from becoming the new norm. Use the SLIP plan below to catch them early, assess the situation, and make a plan for how to proceed. You can also plan to avoid slips by identifying potential triggers and the possible coping plans you can use when you can't avoid the triggers (complete the "My Top Triggers and Coping Plans" portion of this handout).

Slip Plan

STOP

The first step is to stop the problem behavior.

If you have already stopped, congratulate yourself.

It may sound silly but you can even say "STOP" out loud to yourself, or picture a big red stop sign.

LOOK

at the situation realistically.

Step back and ask what you did.

Be specific.

No situation is all or none.

INVESTIGATE

the circumstances.

What kept you from following your plan?

What are other ways you can achieve your goal?

Are your goals specific? Realistic? Achievable?

PROCEED

with your new plan with positive self-talk.

Write down your goals.

Build in some rewards for achieving them.

Get moving on them!

I am confident because

1. **I have these strengths:** _____

2. **I have practiced these things:** _____

_____

3. **I was already able to make these changes:** _____

_____

(continued)

Steps I can take to avoid slips and get back on track as soon as possible:

1. Avoid triggers when possible.
2. Make a coping plan for each trigger and use it when I can't avoid the trigger.

My top triggers and coping plans:

Trigger #1: _____

How I can avoid it: _____

_____

_____

How I plan to cope when I can't avoid it: _____

_____

_____

Trigger #2: _____

How I can avoid it: _____

_____

_____

How I plan to cope when I can't avoid it: _____

_____

_____

Trigger #3: _____

How I can avoid it: _____

_____

_____

How I plan to cope when I can't avoid it: _____

_____

_____

Trigger #4: _____

How I can avoid it: _____

_____

_____

How I plan to cope when I can't avoid it: _____

_____

_____

Change Plan for Maintenance

My Plan

Changes I would like to maintain:

_____

_____

_____

_____

Maintaining these changes is important to me because:

_____

_____

_____

_____

I plan to keep doing these things to maintain my changes (what, where, when, how):

_____

_____

_____

_____

_____

IF this gets in the way	THEN try this
_____	_____
_____	_____
_____	_____
_____	_____
_____	_____
_____	_____
_____	_____

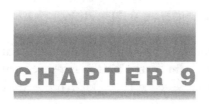

CHAPTER 9

Using This Book as
an Integrated Treatment Manual

This book is based on the premise that there are general relational factors shared among psychosocial treatments and that they account for a significant amount of treatment success beyond specific intervention techniques. We presented how MI provides a framework for these relational factors and specifies skills (e.g., reflections, open questions, ATA) to ensure that these factors are actually present in treatment sessions. We then demonstrated how these same skills are utilized across shared elements of CBT.

"Shared elements" refer to the components of evidence-based clinical practice that are common across distinct treatment protocols. In this book, we presented how the shared elements of CBT (assessment; self-monitoring; between-session practice; cognitive, behavioral, and emotional regulation skills training; and maintenance of change) are integrated with MI to address a wide range of concerns from substance use to health behaviors to internalizing symptoms. In this way, this book provides a universal, evidence-based approach to behavior change and symptom remission. By identifying relational factors and shared elements among CBT approaches and applying them across different areas of behavior change (with specific adaptation for symptom clusters as necessary), we increase the reach of evidence-based treatments while simplifying implementation and training.

> A universal, evidence-based approach to behavior change and symptom remission.

Our integrative approach fits with recent interest in "transdiagnostic" or "unified" treatments that aim to reduce the expense, training, and time needed to master disorder-specific evidence-based CBT protocols (McEvoy et al., 2009).

An Integrated Treatment Manual

Some transdiagnostic treatments utilize a single unified protocol across conditions, while others take a modular approach (McHugh, Murray, & Barlow, 2009). Modular treatment approaches are structured so that not all modules have to be administered to all clients, and the "dose" of each module can be tailored to the individual needs of the patient. We propose that the four MI processes (engaging, focusing, evoking, planning) and associated MI skills (reflections, questions, and ATA) form the core principles for an integrated treatment and that the chapter structure of this text, based on the shared elements of CBT, can be used as an integrated modular treatment manual:

- Module 1: Initial Motivational Session (Chapter 2).
- Module 2: Assessment and Treatment Planning (Chapter 3).
- Module 3: Self-Monitoring (Chapter 4).
- Module 4: Cognitive Skills (Chapter 5).
- Module 5: Skills Training (including problem-solving skills, behavioral activation, distress tolerance, mindfulness and relaxation with or without exposure, refusal skills and assertiveness training, communication skills, organization and planning skills; Chapter 6).
- Module 6: Maintenance of Change (Chapter 8).

The practitioner is encouraged to be flexible in how he or she orders the processes and not feel compelled to cover all four processes in every session. Following the initial motivational session, each session may be structured as follows:

- Discuss session agenda.
- Check in on previous week including assessment of outcomes (e.g., reviewing change plan and homework completion, administering objective measures if applicable).
- Complete brief functional analysis of change or lack thereof.
- Discuss rationales for treatment element or module.
- Elicit and reinforce change talk for behavior change and session tasks.
- Complete session tasks (including expert modeling, guided practice, behavioral rehearsal, and feedback for skills).
- Develop change plan (including implementation intentions, if–then plans, and between-session practice).

Case Examples

To demonstrate how the proposed integrated MI–CBT treatment can be utilized for many different target behaviors or concerns, consider the following additional case examples of problems distinct from those articulated by our prior cases.

Gambling and Anger Management

This first case combines addiction with emotional regulation concerns. Because the data are not clear whether sequential versus simultaneous behavior change is preferable, we allow the client to choose the approach.

Presenting Concern

Antonio is a 32-year-old multiracial man who lives in an urban area with his wife, who is expecting their first child in 4 months. He is recently unemployed, having been terminated from his job as an automotive sales manager after an altercation with the general manager. Assault and battery charges were filed against him, and he was ordered by the court to receive treatment for anger management. His wife urged him to receive treatment for his gambling problem too, since gambling resulted in the foreclosure of their house and repossession of their car in the last 2 years. She threatened to leave him if he could not control his anger and gambling before the birth of their baby. His gambling largely consisted of going to the casino and occasionally going to illegal gambling locations to play poker or other card games. His anger most often took the form of verbal aggression, but sometimes included physical aggression directed toward people and objects (e.g., punching the wall). In his initial session, Antonio was emphatic that he did not want be in counseling because he didn't have a problem with gambling or anger, and he could deal with his anger on his own. He blamed his wife and former boss for his anger and gambling, saying that they pressured him too much and tried to control his life; however, he said that he planned to attend all sessions because he did not want to lose his wife and baby or go to jail. Additionally, he wanted to be able to get another job, house, and car, and he thought that attending treatment might be one way that he could reach his goals.

Functional Assessment and Treatment Planning

A functional assessment of Antonio's gambling and anger was completed as part of treatment planning (see Figure 9.1). Antonio's priorities for both gambling and anger were to avoid people and places that were triggers for him, and to reduce his stress. Antonio chose to work on gambling and anger simultaneously, reasoning that there is a close relationship between the two, and he was prepared to address

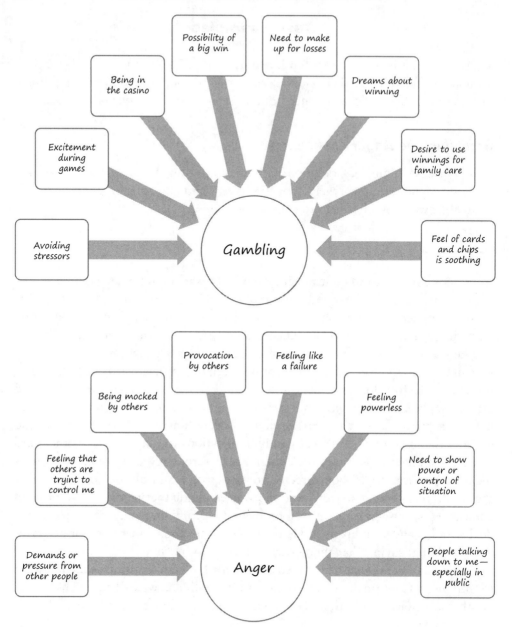

FIGURE 9.1. Functional assessment of Antonio's target behaviors/concerns.

both. Figure 9.2 demonstrates the treatment plan and change talk, and Table 9.1 shows sessions delivered and relevant chapters.

Outcomes

• Antonio attended 90% of all sessions and completed approximately 75% of his between-session practice assignments. He did not have any gambling relapses during treatment. He did have two episodes of verbal aggression that did not escalate to physical aggression, and both episodes occurred before Session 10.

• At the time of discharge, he had met his goals of maintaining his family relationships and staying out of jail. Additionally, he completed a vocational rehabilitation program and entered a debt management program offered through a local social services organization.

• Antonio gained better insight into the relationship between his triggers, behaviors (gambling and anger), and maintaining consequences. He expressed

Target Behavior/ Symptom/Concern	Goals and Objectives	Treatment Plan
1. Gambling	a. Avoid triggers whenever possible b. Develop a coping plan to be used when triggers cannot be avoided c. Use stress management techniques to prevent gambling as a reaction to stress	1a. Self-monitoring; trigger avoidance 1b. Coping skills training; cognitive restructuring 1c. Relaxation: progressive muscle relaxation; mindfulness training
2. Anger	a. Avoid triggers whenever possible b. Develop a coping plan to be used when triggers cannot be avoided c. Avoid verbal and physical aggression as a reaction to stress	2a. Self-monitoring; trigger avoidance; exposure and respotnse prevention 2b. Coping skills training; cognitive restructuring 2c. Distress tolerance; Relaxation: progressive muscle relaxation; mindfulness training

Three reasons why this plan is important to me:

1. *I don't want to lose my wife and baby.*
2. *I don't want to go to jail.*
3. *I want to be able to get another job, house, and car.*

FIGURE 9.2. Antonio's treatment plan.

TABLE 9.1. Antonio's Sessions

Module	Session No.	Relevant Chapter
Initial Motivation Session	1	Chapter 2
Assessment and Treatment Planning	2–3	Chapter 3
Self-Monitoring	4–5	Chapter 4
Skills Training: Problem-Solving Triggers	6–7	Chapter 6
Skills Training for Gambling: Refusal Skills	8–9	Chapter 6
Skills Training for Anger: Assertiveness and Communication Skills Training	10–11	Chapter 6
Cognitive Skills for Gambling	12	Chapter 5
Booster Motivation Session[a]	13	Chapter 2
Cognitive Skills for Anger	14	Chapter 5
Exposure and Response Prevention for Anger	15–18	Chapter 6
Distress Tolerance: Muscle Relaxation	19	Chapter 6
Mindfulness	20–21	Chapter 6
Maintenance and Termination	22–25	Chapter 8

[a]Antonio expressed significant discord in Session 13 and resentment toward his wife and boss for having to attend therapy sessions. Antonio and his counselor postponed the planned cognitive restructuring session and engaged in an MI session focused on reducing discord.

gratitude to his counselor at the end of treatment for being compassionate and accepting throughout treatment while helping him to recognize how to better manage his impulses.

Chronic Cancer Pain and Depression

This next example addresses typical issues in pain management, difficulties with adherence to medications, and concurrent depressed mood. Both MI and CBT have been recommended for self-management of pain, targeting both adherence to medications and adherence to other pain management techniques (e.g., relaxation) (Dorflinger, Kerns, & Auerbach, 2013). MI alone has reduced depressive symptoms in chronic illness and other somatic populations (Naar & Flynn, 2015). Addressing pain management first with an MI foundation may alleviate some of the depressed mood.

Presenting Concern

Lorna is a 46-year-old Caucasian woman with chronic pain post-breast cancer treatment including surgery, and depression following breast cancer diagnosis and treatment 2 years ago. She is in remission following surgery, chemotherapy, and radiation therapy; however, she continues to experience neuropathy, fatigue, and limited mobility in her arms as a result of the cancer treatment. She lives in a rural town with her husband and two sons, ages 13 and 17 years, and transportation to medical providers is difficult for her. Her family is supportive, but their relationships with Lorna have been strained by heavy caregiver responsibilities in the past 2 years, and subsequently the time they have spent together has been less than enjoyable. Additionally, her self-worth has suffered as a result of appearance concerns now that she has had both breasts removed and did not get reconstructive surgery because it was not covered by her medical plan. One of her goals is for her family to enjoy spending time with her again. She is unemployed and was receiving state disability benefits until 2 months ago. Her benefits eligibility was terminated following her recertification when the assessment concluded that she could return to work. Lorna has recently been preoccupied by financial distress and concern that she will not be able to return to work as her pain is not well controlled. In addition to improving her family relationships, Lorna wants to improve her quality of life, and she wants to love herself again.

Lorna was referred by her physician for outpatient therapy for depression and pain management. Her physician also referred her to a physical therapist and a pain specialist. She refused physical therapy due to issues with transportation and the perception that it would not help, but has been able to make appointments with her pain specialist once a month for the past 4 months. At this time, she is prescribed OxyContin (20 mg every 12 hours, tablet form). She is concerned that her pain has not been adequately relieved. Consultation with Dr. Perry, the pain specialist, reveals that Lorna is nonadherent to her medication regimen, often missing doses or taking them at incorrect times. This is because she feels that she "should not" be taking OxyContin, and also because it causes gastrointestinal (GI) problems/constipation. She does not adhere to recommendations for stool softeners. She also does not practice the relaxation techniques that the nurse had showed her. Dr. Perry believes that improving her adherence will allow her medication dose to be properly evaluated and adjusted such that she obtains significant pain relief rather than simply increasing the dose. Supplementing with other self-management techniques could have a synergistic effect.

Lorna was skeptical that counseling would help to reduce her pain, and she returned to this idea many times throughout treatment.

Functional Assessment and Treatment Planning

A functional assessment of chronic cancer pain and depression was conducted as part of treatment planning (see Figure 9.3). Lorna's priorities were to reduce her pain so that she could return to work. She agreed to work on improving her medication adherence in order to determine whether it would make her pain more

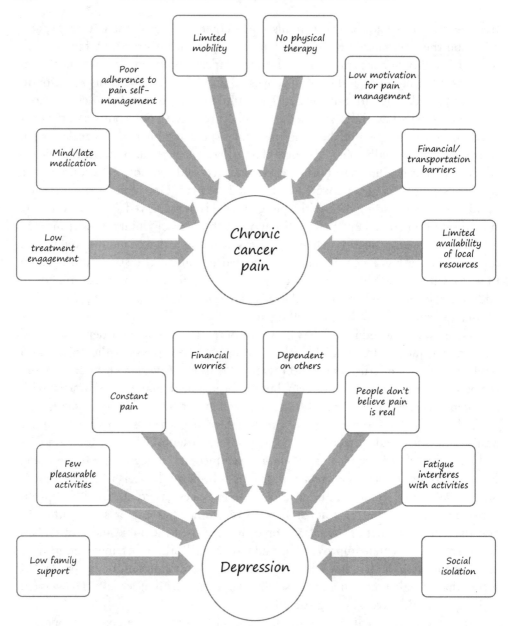

FIGURE 9.3. Functional assessment of Lorna's behaviors/concerns.

tolerable. She also agreed that physical therapy could potentially help with pain management, but she did not think that she could attend appointments regularly because of transportation and financial barriers. She was given a social work referral to address these barriers and she agreed to consider physical therapy if she could work on planning and organization to manage appointments. Lorna did not feel hopeful that she could reduce her depression unless her pain was controlled. Thus, she chose to work on pain management and depression sequentially. She agreed to try behavior activation via a pacing approach after addressing her pain management. Her other priorities were to increase social support, and worry less about whether others believed that her pain was real or not. Figure 9.4 demonstrates the treatment plan and change talk, and Table 9.2 shows sessions delivered and relevant chapters.

Target Behavior/Symptom/Concern	Goals and Objectives	Treatment Plan
1. Chronic cancer pain	a. Reduce pain to no more than 1 day per week with a pain rating above 5 (on 0–10 scale) b. Return to part-time work within 2 months (discontinued)	1a. Medication adherence: self-monitoring; planning and organization skills 1b. Distress tolerance: mindfulness training; progressive muscle relaxation 1c. Attend physical therapy
2. Feeling depressed	a. Do at least one pleasurable activity every day b. Increase supportive contact with others to at least three contacts per week (with at least one away from home) c. Replace worries about whether others believe pain is real with helpful thoughts	2a. Behavioral activation: self-monitoring; activity scheduling 2b. Communication skills to build social support: assess needs and resources, build a social support plan; communication skills 2c. Worries about others' beliefs: cognitive restructuring

Three reasons why this plan is important to me:

1. *I want to improve my quality of life.*
2. *I want my family to enjoy spending time with me.*
3. *I want to love myself despite the changes in my life that I cannot control.*

FIGURE 9.4. Lorna's treatment plan.

TABLE 9.2. Lorna's Sessions

Module	Session No.	Relevant Chapter
Initial Motivation Session	1	Chapter 2
Assessment and Treatment Planning	2	Chapter 3
Pain Self-Monitoring	3	Chapter 4
Booster Motivation Session for Treatment Engagement[a]	4	Chapter 2
Skills Training for Pain: Planning and Organization	6–7	Chapter 6
Skills Training for Pain: Mindfulness	8–9	Chapter 6
Motivation Booster for Between-Session Practice[b]	10	Chapter 7
Skills Training for Pain: Relaxation	11	Chapter 6
Motivation Booster for Attendance and Depression Focus[c]	12	Chapter 7
Depression: Behavioral Activation	13	Chapters 4 and 6
Behavioral Activation (continued)	14	Chapter 6
Depression: Communication Skills to Build Social Support	15	Chapter 6
Depression: Cognitive Restructuring	16	Chapter 5
Termination Session	17	Chapter 8

[a]Lorna discontinued her goal of returning to work part-time and decided to appeal the termination of her disability benefits. In Session 4, she discussed discontinuing therapy as well. Her therapist postponed the planning and organization session and delivered an MI session focused on reengaging Lorna in treatment.
[b]Lorna had missed her between-session practice for mindfulness following Sessions 8 and 9. The MI session discussed the linkage of success to practice and supporting autonomy. Lorna decided she could incorporate a few mindfulness strategies but wanted to move on to another skill.
[c]After continuing to miss between-session practice following Session 11, Lorna expressed consideration of termination because of lack of optimism in treatment and competing priorities with all of the appointments she had to attend. The counselor reengaged the client with MI skills, and they developed a new focus on depressed mood.

Outcomes

• Lorna attended 85% of her sessions and completed approximately 50% of her between-session practice assignments.

• She obtained case management services through a local social services organization to assist with financial and transportation barriers.

• The number of days with pain ratings above 5 (on a 0–10 scale) was reduced from 7 to 3 days a week, likely due to better medication adherence and starting adjunctive medications for GI side effects. Lorna had a plan to start physical therapy at the end of psychotherapy.

• At least one pleasurable activity was completed 5 days a week.

• Supportive contacts with others increased to at least three per week (with at least one away from home).

- Worries about whether others believed Lorna's pain was real were not appreciably reduced; and she terminated treatment before completing all the treatment tasks related to depression. However, she believed her mood had notably improved over the course of treatment.

- At the time of discharge, Lorna said that she had made satisfactory progress toward achieving each of her goals. She still believed that her pain was not effectively managed, but her improved family relationships, reduced social isolation, and increased pleasurable activities contributed to an improved quality of life. She said that her family was beginning to initiate conversations and activities with her rather than avoiding her, and she was starting to view herself as a loveable person again.

We presented these case examples to illustrate how an integrated MI–CBT approach presented in this book might be applicable to a wide range of presenting problems.

Summary of MI–CBT Dilemmas

The MI–CBT dilemmas presented in the preceding chapters all concern the themes of timing and content of sessions. When do you continue to spend time addressing ambivalence with MI strategies versus moving on with CBT tasks? In MI you would continue with engaging and evoking and potentially not move to planning if the client is not demonstrating sufficient commitment to change. However, ambivalence may not fully resolve before engaging in CBT. You may spend more than a session or two on building motivation; however, at some point you might suggest moving to try out the next steps in CBT as a behavioral experiment. You may then continue to engage, focus, and evoke motivation for changing target behaviors and for participating in treatment during subsequent CBT sessions when ambivalence interferes with progression.

What do you do when the client's preference for treatment content runs counter to the evidence of what is effective (what clients want vs. what clients need)? Consider the following choices. You may inform the client about what is necessary for the CBT you provide (using ATA) and if the client is not ready to complete the task, then the client may not be ready for CBT. You may decide to see the client for MI-only sessions or to have him or her return to see you when he or she is ready to engage in what you consider to be a necessary treatment ingredient. Alternatively, you can decide to provide MI–CBT without that treatment ingredient, perhaps asking the client to reconsider if progress is not sufficient. Finally, you may try to negotiate alternatives to the treatment ingredient. What would you do? The choice is not always clear; however, following this approach, it can be helpful to maintain collaboration with the client, and any decisions about either moving on without a treatment component, terminating, taking a break, or continuing to work on motivation to resolve ambivalence should be explicit.

Training in MI–CBT Integration

Research on how to effectively train practitioners in MI and CBT as stand-alone treatments is beginning to emerge (Barwick, Bennett, Johnson, McGowan, & Moore, 2012), but studies on training in MI–CBT integration are practically non-existent. To the best of our knowledge, the only publications on this topic come from the COMBINE trial, a combined MI and CBT intervention targeting alcohol use (Anton et al., 2006). Miller and colleagues (2005) reported on the process of training and quality monitoring. First, they chose to screen practitioners for a pre-requisite level of proficiency in accurate empathy, by rating two 10-minute practice tapes with an objective coding scheme (Moyers, Martin, Catley, Harris, & Ahlu-walia, 2003), in the hopes of shortening the time required to be proficient in MI. In advance of the initial 7-day workshop, practitioners were instructed to read a text on MI and the treatment manual. They reviewed six training videos on MI and three on CBT. Practitioners then submitted recordings of all of the MI–CBT treatment sessions for two clients, which were coded with a session checklist that included MI components and CBT components. The coding recorded whether the treatment element was present but not the quality of the treatment element.

There is limited information on how available MI fidelity coding schemes may be used to code the quality of MI within CBT sessions when MI and CBT are integrated, though Moyers and colleagues have coded a variety of treatment sessions in Project MATCH, a study comparing MI, CBT, and 12-step treatments for alcohol (Moyers et al., 2007). They found that across treatment approaches, client change talk was related to behavior change in substance use, though counselors' MI skill was not coded in the CBT and 12-step sessions. These data suggest that the relationship between client language and treatment outcomes is also seen in therapeutic approaches other than MI, suggesting that evoking change talk may be a common mechanism of outcome across treatment approaches.

We have preliminary data on a rating scale for MI fidelity within sessions where practitioners are expected to integrate MI and CBT. In a small pilot study, supervisors rated counselors on MI components using a 4-point rating scale. The preliminary results from measurement models (Chapman, Sheidow, Henggeler, Halliday-Boykins, & Cunningham, 2008) are promising: the components formed a single dimension; the 4-point rating scale performed as intended; the components assessed the full range of counselors and families; and the components could dif-ferentiate about five levels of MI fidelity in the sample. The final MI fidelity mea-sure (Naar & Flynn, 2015) is presented in Table 9.3 and is currently being used in several federally funded projects.

TABLE 9.3. Measure of MI Fidelity in CBT Sessions: The MI Coach Rating Scale

Item	Definition
1. The counselor cultivates empathy and compassion with the client.	The counselor understands or makes an effort to grasp the client's perspective and feelings, and convey that understanding to the client.
2. The counselor fosters collaboration with the client.	The counselor negotiates with the client and avoids an authoritarian stance. A metaphor for collaboration is dancing instead of wrestling.
3. The counselor supports autonomy of the client.	The counselor emphasizes the client's freedom of choice and conveys an understanding that the critical variables for change are within the client him- or herself and cannot be imposed by others.
4. The counselor works to evoke the client's ideas and motivations for change.	The counselor conveys an understanding that motivation for change, and the ability to move toward that change, reside mostly within the client and therefore focuses efforts to elicit and expand it within the therapeutic interaction.
5. The counselor balances the client's agenda with focusing on the target behaviors.	The counselor maintains appropriate focus on a specific target behavior or concerns directly tied to it while still addressing the client's concerns.
6. The counselor demonstrates reflective listening skills.	The frequency of reflective statements is in balance with questions.
7. The counselor uses reflections strategically.	Low-quality reflections are inaccurate, lengthy, or unclear; high-quality reflections are used to express empathy, develop discrepancy, reinforce change talk, reduce resistance, and generally strategically to increase motivation.
8. The counselor reinforces strengths and positive behavior change with affirmations/ affirming reflections.	The counselor affirms personal qualities or efforts made by the client that promote productive change or that the client might harness in future change efforts.
9. The counselor uses summaries effectively.	Summaries are used to pull together points from two or more prior client statements. At least two different ideas must be conveyed, as opposed to two reflections of the same idea. Summaries are a way to express active listening and reflect back to the client the "story." Summaries are also used to structure the session as well as to guide the client in the direction of change.
10. The counselor asks questions in an open-ended way.	An open-ended question is one that allows a wide range of possible answers. Closed-ended questions may be answered with a one-word response. Multiple-choice questions are considered open, particularly with clients who struggle with open and more abstract questions.
11. The counselor solicits feedback from the client.	The counselor asks the client for his or her response to information, recommendations, feedback, etc. This is analogous to the ask–tell–ask or elicit–provide–elicit strategy in MI.
12. The counselor manages counterchange talk/sustain talk and discord.	The counselor responds to discord and sustain talk (i.e., counterchange talk) either reflectively or strategically. The client may make statements against change either directly about the target behaviors, about engaging in the treatment program, or about discord in the relationship. Discord refers to tension between the client and the counselor (wrestling).

We know little about how to train MI practitioners in CBT or how to train CBT practitioners in MI. The COMBINE trial trained new practitioners with a foundation in accurate empathy in MI–CBT integration, but the content of training was not published. Our own experience with training MI–CBT integration used Miller and Rollnick (2013) as a foundation. Table 9.4 proposes a possible plan for training new practitioners in MI–CBT integration so that integration is taught up front instead of later. See *behaviorchangeconsulting.org* for more information about training in MI-CBT and the MI-CBT fidelity measure.

Emerging Issues

Multiple Health Behavior Change and Comorbidity

In the last decade, there has been an increasing focus on changing multiple behaviors because many co-occur and covary (Prochaska, Spring, & Nigg, 2008). Targeting two or more related behaviors may increase providers' ability to help individuals make more meaningful changes with fewer costs and resources than if each behavior was targeted separately (Prochaska et al., 2008). A 2011 review found only four studies that directly compared simultaneous and sequential approaches to multiple behavior change (Prochaska & Prochaska, 2011). Three studies targeted tobacco and diet (Spring et al., 2004), tobacco and alcohol (Joseph, Willenbring, Nugent, & Nelson, 2004), and physical activity and diet (Vandelanotte, De Bourdeaudhuij, Sallis, Spittaels, & Brug, 2005). There were no differences between simultaneous versus sequential interventions on long-term outcomes. In one study targeting physical activity, tobacco, and sodium, the simultaneous intervention was superior to the sequential intervention (Hyman, Pavlik, Taylor, Goodrick, &

TABLE 9.4. Training Plan for MI–CBT Integration

Step 1.	MI spirit and MI skills (reflections, open questions, ATA).
Step 2.	Engaging process; practice engaging in the context of setting session agenda.
Step 3.	Focusing process; practice focusing in the context of treatment planning.
Step 4.	Evoking process; practice evoking in the context of discussing rationale for self-monitoring.
Step 5.	Planning process; practice planning in the context of self-monitoring assignments.
Step 6.	Pulling together all four processes in the initial session.
Step 7.	Pulling together all four processes in cognitive-behavioral skills-building sessions.

Moye, 2007). Most of the studies utilized skills-building interventions but not necessarily MI. However, in synthesis of meta-analyses and reviews of physical activity and nutrition target behaviors, single behavioral treatments (activity-only or nutrition-only) were superior to interventions targeting both simultaneously (Sweet & Fortier, 2010). We found one additional study published since that review (King et al., 2013) comparing simultaneous targeting of nutrition and physical activity with two sequential plans—physical activity first and nutrition first—and a control condition matched for length of treatment. After 4 months

> Targeting two or more related behaviors will help you help clients make more meaningful changes.

of treatment, the physical activity-first condition resulted in greater changes in activity compared to the other three conditions. Both sequential and simultaneous interventions were better than the control condition in changing nutrition. However, long-term outcomes (12 months) were not different by condition, with one exception. The nutrition-first sequential condition seemed to suppress physical activity changes; thus the authors recommended a simultaneous approach based on the findings overall.

Similar concerns arise when treating comorbid conditions (Mueser & Drake, 2007). Options include sequential treatment, parallel treatment, and integrated treatments (Ries, 1996). Historically, sequential treatment has been the most common, and in the case of comorbid mental health and substance abuse conditions, the patient may engage in one treatment system and then the other with separate treatments and practitioners. In the parallel treatment approach, treatments are provided separately but simultaneously. If different practitioners are providing treatments, adequate coordination becomes especially critical. Integrated treatment is also simultaneous, but both conditions are treated by the same practitioner and the interrelationship between conditions is explicitly addressed. The same treatment strategies may be used to target similar symptom clusters. Again there is limited data on the best approach.

Clinically, we have found that if the target behaviors have similar antecedents based on functional analysis, it may be beneficial to target them simultaneously. However, some clients feel overwhelmed trying to make too many behavior changes at once. Until the data clearly suggest how to address multiple behavior change, we believe the best approach is to allow the client to choose as part of collaborative treatment planning by providing a menu of options.

Acceptance and Commitment Therapy and MI

Acceptance and commitment therapy (ACT; Hayes, Strosahl, & Wilson, 2012) is perhaps the most studied treatment of the "third-wave" of behavioral (first-wave) and cognitive-behavioral (second-wave) therapies. Third-wave therapies focus on changing the function of psychological events, rather than on changing or modifying the events themselves (Hayes, 2004). (Note that dialectical behavior therapy is sometimes referred to as second wave and sometimes as third wave, and thus was included in Chapter 6.) The goals of ACT are to increase the ability to mindfully be present in the moment and to engage in behaviors that serve core values. These goals are achieved through six core ACT processes: acceptance, cognitive defusion (accepting negative thoughts vs. restructuring), being present, self as context (observing the world vs. interpreting), chosen values, and committed action. The most recent meta-analysis (Davis, Morina, Powers, Smits, & Emmelkamp, 2015) of 39 randomized controlled trials suggested that ACT was more effective than waitlist and treatment as usual.

When we focused on integrating MI with shared elements of CBT, we did not specifically include ACT, although mindfulness is addressed as a skill in Chapter 6. Bricker and Tollison (2011) compared the conceptualization and clinical strategies of MI and ACT. MI focuses on the content of language (e.g., change talk vs. counterchange talk), whereas ACT focuses on the processes of language that are involved in pathology (e.g., how language is used to interpret context). However, the similarities suggest that integration is feasible. Similarities include a focus on enhancing commitment to behavior change, using client's values to enhance commitment, and to work with client's language to achieve these goals. Further trials and clinical case studies are needed to specify this integration and demonstrate efficacy.

Using Extrinsic Reinforcers

Though MI centers on developing of intrinsic motivation, some behavior change interventions focus on the systematic utilization of incentives such as vouchers for clean urine tests or weight loss, token economies, and family behavior plans. There is some concern that the use of extrinsic reinforcers can undermine intrinsic motivation. However, investigations about intrinsic and extrinsic motivation have shown these to be separate phenomena, and not inversely related (Lepper, Corpus, & Iyengar, 2005). Others researchers have pointed to the additive effect of intrinsic and extrinsic motivational approaches (i.e., targeting internal motivators, such as achievement of personal goals, and simultaneously using external motivators, such as offering monetary incentives for goal attainment). Targeting both aspects of motivation may have a synergistic effect. The simultaneous use of MI skills along with extrinsic reinforcers can promote the identification of internal reasons for maintaining the new behavior (Carroll & Rounsaville, 2007; Vallerand, 1997).

Extrinsic motivators should be offered as a menu of options to support autonomy and decrease counterchange talk and discord. Strategies related to evoking can be used to elicit and reinforce change talk and solidify commitment throughout extrinsic motivation to increase the internalization of motivation. Examples of counselor statements that might be heard in such a treatment would be: "I know you say that right now you are only doing this to get off probation. What would life be like if you continued this behavior change?" or "You completed 30 minutes of exercise so you could get your prize and you said that you felt stronger when you did it. How does that fit with what you said about being a strong, independent person?" In this way, the extrinsic reinforcement begins to tip the scale of ambivalence. MI strategies may support the maintenance of initial changes by promoting intrinsic motivation. Few studies have addressed the best way to integrate MI with extrinsic reinforcement approaches such as contingency management, though there is some evidence that combined approaches are efficacious (Carroll et al., 2006; Naar-King et al., 2016).

Using Technology to Deliver MI–CBT Integrated Treatments

The last decade has seen a burgeoning of technology-delivered behavioral interventions. Meta-analyses reviewing computer-delivered CBT suggest efficacy compared to no treatment control conditions (Adelman, Panza, Bartley, Bontempo, & Bloch, 2014; Ebert et al., 2015). However, these data are certainly limited by not having comparisons to in-person approaches, and a common element of integrated MI–CBT is the relational component. Several studies have demonstrated the efficacy of computer-delivered MI (Kiene & Barta, 2006; Naar-King, Outlaw, et al., 2013; Ondersma, Chase, Svikis, & Schuster, 2005; Ondersma et al., 2012; Ondersma, Svikis, & Schuster, 2007; Ondersma, Svikis, Thacker, Beatty, & Lockhart, 2014; Schwartz et al., 2014; Tzilos, Sokol, & Ondersma, 2011), but with limited studies comparing computer-delivered with face-to-face treatments. Using technology to deliver MI–CBT integrated treatments has not yet been fully studied and is an area for future research, though several of the MI studies included CBT strategies such as behavioral skills.

Final Words

Integrated (unified or transdiagnostic) treatments may be the wave of the future, but how to best learn MI, CBT, and its integration is not yet fully known. Learning a new treatment can be like learning a new language. Is the goal of learning MI–CBT to be bilingual or is the goal for MI–CBT to be a new language in and of itself? When you are fluent in two languages, one language may be primary because it was learned first and spoken more often, but the other has been learned to help you navigate new contexts. In linguistics, the term "code switching" refers to alternating between two languages in a single conversation (Milroy & Muysken, 1995). More recently, linguists (Auer, 1999) distinguish code mixing as the convergence of two languages into a "fused lect," a relatively stable mixed language such as "Spanglish." We believe this fused lect comes closer to MI–CBT integration. Regardless of whether you feel you are code switching or code mixing, it is clear that bilingualism has advantages in many cognitive domains (Adescope, Lavin, Thompson, & Ungerleider, 2010).

If there is one golden rule in learning a new language or languages, we believe it is "practice." Reviewing training exercises and practicing them alone or in a peer group can be particularly helpful. Observing practitioners deliver MI–CBT can be an excellent model for learning (Moyers videos for COMBINE). Listening to and coding your own or your peers' recordings for MI and CBT competency can enhance your knowledge. While integrated MI–CBT coding schemes are rare, you may code the same sessions for MI competency and CBT competency. We have noted at least two coding schemes for MI that seem to work for CBT sessions including the MITI (*http://casaa.unm.edu/download/MITI4_2.pdf*), checklists from the COMBINE trial (*www.cscc.unc.edu/combine/procman/CBIManual032802.pdf*), and the MI Coach Rating Scale (Table 9.3), and one published of fidelity to an MI–CBT integrated treatment (Haddock ct al., 2012).

> The golden rule in learning a new language: "practice."

Recall that practice over time with guided feedback is the key to becoming proficient, and this mantra applies even once you are well down the path of having learned how to integrate MI and CBT. After reading this text, you may continue your own journey of change including workshop attendance, coaching and supervision, review of session recordings, peer supervision, and most importantly listening to the talk of young people. These are all paths to learning MI–CBT integration. Which one will you choose next?

━━━━━━━━━━━ **ACTIVITY 9.1 FOR PRACTITIONERS** ━━━━━━━━━━━

Your Change Plan for MI–CBT Integration

We provided a menu of options for training yourself in MI–CBT integration including studying this text, attending a workshop, reviewing recordings of MI–CBT sessions, coding your own recordings, and possibly training others in MI–CBT. Consider developing your own change plan for continuing your journey in MI–CBT integration.

ACTIVITY GOAL: This activity supports the planning process for your own skill development in delivering MI–CBT integration.

ACTIVITY INSTRUCTIONS: Complete the following change plan and share with a colleague.

My Change Plan

Changes I would like to make to deliver MI–CBT:

_____
_____
_____
_____

These changes are important to me because:

_____
_____
_____
_____

I plan to take these steps (what, where, when, how):

_____
_____
_____
_____

IF this gets in the way	**THEN try this**

References

Abraham, C., & Michie, S. (2008). A taxonomy of behavior change techniques used in interventions. *Health Psychology, 27*(3), 379–387.

Addis, M. E., & Carpenter, K. M. (2000). The treatment rationale in cognitive behavioral therapy: Psychological mechanisms and clinical guidelines. *Cognitive and Behavioral Practice, 7*(2), 147–156.

Adelman, C. B., Panza, K. E., Bartley, C. A., Bontempo, A., & Bloch, M. H. (2014). A meta-analysis of computerized cognitive-behavioral therapy for the treatment of DSM-5 anxiety disorders. *Journal of Clinical Psychiatry, 75*(7), e695–e704.

Adescope, O. O., Lavin, T., Thompson, T., & Ungerleider, C. (2010). A systematic review and meta-analysis of the cognitive correlates of bilingualism. *Review of Educational Research, 80*(2), 207–245.

Amati, F., Barthassat, V., Miganne, G., Hausman, I., Monnin, D. G., Costanza, M. C., et al. (2007). Enhancing regular physical activity and relapse prevention through a 1-day therapeutic patient education workshop: A pilot study. *Patient Education and Counseling, 68*(1), 70–78.

Anderson, E. S., Wojcik, J. R., Winett, R. A., & Williams, D. M. (2006). Social-cognitive determinants of physical activity: The influence of social support, self-efficacy, outcome expectations, and self-regulation among participants in a church-based health promotion study. *Health Psychology, 25*(4), 510–520.

Andersson, E. K., & Moss, T. P. (2011). Imagery and implementation intention: A randomised controlled trial of interventions to increase exercise behaviour in the general population. *Psychology of Sport and Exercise, 12*(2), 63–70.

Anton, R. F., O'Malley, S. S., Ciraulo, D. A., Cisler, R. A., Couper, D., Donovan, D. M., et al. (2006). Combined pharmacotherapies and behavioral interventions for alcohol dependence: The COMBINE study: A randomized controlled trial. *Journal of the American Medical Association, 295*(17), 2003–2017.

221

Auer, P. (1999). From codeswitching via language mixing to fused lects toward a dynamic typology of bilingual speech. *International Journal of Bilingualism, 3*(4), 309–332.

Babor, T. F. (2004). Brief treatments for cannabis dependence: Findings from a randomized multisite trial. *Journal of Consulting and Clinical Psychology, 72*(3), 455–466.

Bandura, A. (2004). Health promotion by social cognitive means. *Health Education and Behavior, 31*(2), 143–164.

Barkley, R. A. (Ed.). (2015). *Attention-deficit hyperactivity disorder: A handbook for diagnosis and treatment* (4th ed.). New York: Guilford Press.

Barth, R. P., Lee, B. R., Lindsey, M. A., Collins, K. S., Strieder, F., Chorpita, B. F., et al. (2012). Evidence-based practice at a crossroads: The timely emergence of common elements and common factors. *Research on Social Work Practice, 22*(1), 108–119.

Barwick, M. A., Bennett, L. M., Johnson, S. N., McGowan, J., & Moore, J. E. (2012). Training health and mental health professionals in motivational interviewing: A systematic review. *Children and Youth Services Review, 34*(9), 1786–1795.

Beck, J. S. (2011). *Cognitive behavior therapy: Basics and beyond* (2nd ed.). New York: Guilford Press.

Bell, A. C., & D'Zurilla, T. J. (2009). Problem-solving therapy for depression: A meta-analysis. *Clinical Psychology Review, 29*(4), 348–353.

Berking, M., Meier, C., & Wupperman, P. (2010). Enhancing emotion-regulation skills in police officers: Results of a pilot controlled study. *Behavior Therapy, 41*(3), 329–339.

Berking, M., & Whitley, B. (2014). Emotion regulation: Definition and relevance for mental health. In *Affect regulation training; A practitioner's manual* (pp. 5–17). New York: Springer.

Beshai, S., Dobson, K. S., Bockting, C. L., & Quigley, L. (2011). Relapse and recurrence prevention in depression: Current research and future prospects. *Clinical Psychology Review, 31*(8), 1349–1360.

Bickel, W. K., & Mueller, E. T. (2009). Toward the study of trans-disease processes: A novel approach with special reference to the study of co-morbidity. *Journal of Dual Diagnosis, 5*(2), 131–138.

Bird, V., Premkumar, P., Kendall, T., Whittington, C., Mitchell, J., & Kuipers, E. (2010). Early intervention services, cognitive-behavioural therapy and family intervention in early psychosis: Systematic review. *British Journal of Psychiatry, 197*(5), 350–356.

Bordin, E. S. (1979). The generalizability of the psychoanalytic concept of the working alliance. *Psychotherapy: Theory, Research and Practice, 16*(3), 252–260.

Borkovec, T. D., Wilkinson, L., Folensbee, R., & Lerman, C. (1983). Stimulus control applications to the treatment of worry. *Behaviour Research and Therapy, 21*(3), 247–251.

Brehm, J. W. (1966). *A theory of psychological reactance.* New York: Academic Press.

Bricker, J., & Tollison, S. (2011). Comparison of motivational interviewing with acceptance and commitment therapy: A conceptual and clinical review. *Behavioural and Cognitive Psychotherapy, 39*(5), 541–559.

Burke, L. E., Wang, J., & Sevick, M. A. (2011). Self-monitoring in weight loss: A systematic review of the literature. *Journal of the American Dietetic Association, 111*(1), 92–102.

Carroll, K. M., Easton, C. J., Nich, C., Hunkele, K. A., Neavins, T. M., Sinha, R., et al. (2006). The use of contingency management and motivational/skills-building therapy to treat young adults with marijuana dependence. *Journal of Consulting and Clinical Psychology, 74*(5), 955–966.

Carroll, K. M., & Rounsaville, B. J. (2007). A vision of the next generation of behavioral therapies research in the addictions. *Addiction, 102*(6), 850–862.

Chapman, J. E., Sheidow, A. J., Henggeler, S. W., Halliday-Boykins, C. A., & Cunningham, P. B. (2008). Developing a measure of therapist adherence to contingency management: An application of the Many-Facet Rasch Model. *Journal of Child and Adolescent Substance Abuse, 17*(3), 47–68.

Chasteen, A. L., Park, D. C., & Schwarz, N. (2001). Implementation intentions and facilitation of prospective memory. *Psychological Science, 12*(6), 457–461.

Chen, J., Liu, X., Rapee, R. M., & Pillay, P. (2013). Behavioural activation: A pilot trial of transdiagnostic treatment for excessive worry. *Behaviour Research and Therapy, 51*(9), 533–539.

Chiesa, A., Calati, R., & Serretti, A. (2011). Does mindfulness training improve cognitive abilities?: A systematic review of neuropsychological findings. *Clinical Psychology Review, 31*(3), 449–464.

Chiesa, A., & Serretti, A. (2009). Mindfulness-based stress reduction for stress management in healthy people: A review and meta-analysis. *Journal of Alternative and Complementary Medicine, 15*(5), 593–600.

Chorpita, B. F., Becker, K. D., Daleiden, E. L., & Hamilton, J. D. (2007). Understanding the common elements of evidence-based practice. *Journal of the American Academy of Child and Adolescent Psychiatry, 46*(5), 647–652.

Connors, G. J., Walitzer, K. S., & Dermen, K. H. (2002). Preparing clients for alcoholism treatment: Effects on treatment participation and outcomes. *Journal of Consulting and Clinical Psychology, 70*(5), 1161–1169.

Craske, M. G., & Barlow, D. H. (2006). *Mastery of your anxiety and panic: Therapist guide.* New York: Oxford University Press.

Craske, M. G., & Tsao, J. C. (1999). Self-monitoring with panic and anxiety disorders. *Psychological Assessment, 11*(4), 466–479.

Davis, M., Morina, N., Powers, M., Smits, J., & Emmelkamp, P. (2015). A meta-analysis of the efficacy of acceptance and commitment therapy for clinically relevant mental and physical health problems. *Psychotherapy and Psychosomatics, 84*(1), 30–36.

Dimeff, L. A., & Koerner, K. E. (2007). *Dialectical behavior therapy in clinical practice: Applications across disorders and settings.* New York: Guilford Press.

Dimidjian, S., Hollon, S. D., Dobson, K. S., Schmaling, K. B., Kohlenberg, R. J., Addis, M. E., et al. (2006). Randomized trial of behavioral activation, cognitive therapy, and antidepressant medication in the acute treatment of adults with major depression. *Journal of Consulting and Clinical Psychology, 74*(4), 658–670.

Dorflinger, L., Kerns, R. D., & Auerbach, S. M. (2013). Providers' roles in enhancing patients' adherence to pain self management. *Translational Behavioral Medicine, 3*(1), 39–46.

Douaihy, A., Daley, D., Stowell, K., Park, T., Witkiewitz, K., & Marlatt, G. (2007). Relapse prevention: Clinical strategies for substance use disorders. In K. Witkiewitz & A.

Marlatt (Eds.), *Therapist's guide to evidence-based relapse prevention* (pp. 37–73). Burlington, MA: Elsevier.

Driessen, E., & Hollon, S. D. (2011). Motivational interviewing from a cognitive behavioral perspective. *Cognitive and Behavioral Practice, 18*(1), 70–73.

Ebert, D. D., Zarski, A.-C., Christensen, H., Stikkelbroek, Y., Cuijpers, P., Berking, M., et al. (2015). Internet and computer-based cognitive behavioral therapy for anxiety and depression in youth: A meta-analysis of randomized controlled outcome trials. *PLoS ONE, 10*(3), e0119895.

Engle, D. E., & Arkowitz, H. (2006). *Ambivalence in psychotherapy: Facilitating readiness to change.* New York: Guilford Press.

Farrell, J. M., Reiss, N., & Shaw, I. A. (2014). *The schema therapy clinician's guide: A complete resource for building and delivering individual, group and integrated schema mode treatment programs.* West Sussex, UK: Wiley.

Fisher, G. L., & Roget, N. A. (2009). *Encyclopedia of substance abuse prevention, treatment, and recovery.* Thousand Oaks, CA: SAGE.

Fixsen, D. L., Naoom, S. F., Blase, K. A., Friedman, R. M., & Wallace, F. (2009). *Implementation research: A synthesis of the literature.* Tampa: National Implementation Research Network, Louis de la Parte Florida Mental Health Institute, University of South Florida.

Fjorback, L., Arendt, M., Ørnbøl, E., Fink, P., & Walach, H. (2011). Mindfulness-based stress reduction and mindfulness-based cognitive therapy: A systematic review of randomized controlled trials. *Acta Psychiatrica Scandinavica, 124*(2), 102–119.

Flynn, H. A. (2011). Setting the stage for the integration of motivational interviewing with cognitive behavioral therapy in the treatment of depression. *Cognitive and Behavioral Practice, 18*(1), 46–54.

Folkman, S. (Ed.). (2011). *The Oxford handbook of stress, health, and coping.* New York: Oxford University Press.

Freeman, A., & McCluskey, R. (2005). Resistance: Impediments to effective psychotherapy. In A. Freeman (Ed.), *Encyclopedia of cognitive behavior therapy* (pp. 334–340). New York: Springer.

Gilbert, P., & Leahy, R. L. (Eds.). (2007). *The therapeutic relationship in the cognitive behavioral psychotherapies.* Hove, East Sussex, UK: Routledge.

Gollwitzer, P. M. (1999). Implementation intentions: Strong effects of simple plans. *American Psychologist, 54*(7), 493–503.

Gollwitzer, P. M., & Sheeran, P. (2006). Implementation intentions and goal achievement: A meta-analysis of effects and processes. *Advances in Experimental Social Psychology, 38*, 69–119.

Gordon, T. (1970). *Parent effectiveness training.* New York: Wyden Books.

Green, C. A., Polen, M. R., Janoff, S. L., Castleton, D. K., Wisdom, J. P., Vuckovic, N., et al. (2008). Understanding how clinician–patient relationships and relational continuity of care affect recovery from serious mental illness: STARS study results. *Psychiatric Rehabilitation Journal, 32*(1), 9–22.

Greenson, R. R. (1971). The "real" relationship between the patient and the psychoanalyst. In M. Kanzer (Ed.), *The unconscious today* (pp. 213–232). New York: International Universities Press.

Haddock, G., Beardmore, R., Earnshaw, P., Fitzsimmons, M., Nothard, S., Butler, R., et al. (2012). Assessing fidelity to integrated motivational interviewing and CBT therapy for psychosis and substance use: The MI-CBT Fidelity Scale (MI-CTS). *Journal of Mental Health, 21*(1), 38–48.

Havassy, B. E., Hall, S. M., & Wasserman, D. A. (1991). Social support and relapse: Commonalities among alcoholics, opiate users, and cigarette smokers. *Addictive Behaviors, 16*(5), 235–246.

Hayes, S. C. (2004). Acceptance and commitment therapy, relational frame theory, and the third wave of behavioral and cognitive therapies. *Behavior Therapy, 35*(4), 639–665.

Hayes, S. C., Strosahl, K. D., & Wilson, K. G. (2012). *Acceptance and commitment therapy: The process and practice of mindful change* (2nd ed.). New York: Guilford Press.

Heckman, C. J., Egleston, B. L., & Hofmann, M. T. (2010). Efficacy of motivational interviewing for smoking cessation: A systematic review and meta-analysis. *Tobacco Control, 19*(5), 410–416.

Henman, M. J., Butow, P. N., Brown, R. F., Boyle, F., & Tattersall, M. H. N. (2002). Lay constructions of decision-making in cancer. *Psycho-Oncology, 11*(4), 295–306.

Herz, M. I., Lamberti, J. S., Mintz, J., Scott, R., O'Dell, S. P., McCartan, L., et al. (2000). A program for relapse prevention in schizophrenia: A controlled study. *Archives of General Psychiatry, 57*(3), 277–283.

Hettema, J., Steele, J., & Miller, W. R. (2005). Motivational interviewing. *Annual Review of Clinical Psychology 1*(1), 91–111.

Hofmann, S. G., Asnaani, A., Vonk, I. J., Sawyer, A. T., & Fang, A. (2012). The efficacy of cognitive behavioral therapy: A review of meta-analyses. *Cognitive Therapy and Research, 36*(5), 427–440.

Horvath, A. O., Del Re, A., Flückiger, C., & Symonds, D. (2011). Alliance in individual psychotherapy. *Psychotherapy, 48*(1), 9–16.

Humphreys, K., Marx, B., & Lexington, J. (2009). Self-monitoring as a treatment vehicle. In W. T. O'Donohue & J. E. Fisher (Eds.), *General principles and empirically supported techniques of cognitive behavior therapy* (pp. 576–583). Hobocken, NJ: Wiley.

Hyman, D. J., Pavlik, V. N., Taylor, W. C., Goodrick, G. K., & Moye, L. (2007). Simultaneous vs sequential counseling for multiple behavior change. *Archives of Internal Medicine, 167*(11), 1152–1158.

Jacob, J. J., & Isaac, R. (2012). Behavioral therapy for management of obesity. *Indian Journal of Endocrinology and Metabolism, 16*(1), 28–32.

Jacobson, N. S., Dobson, K. S., Truax, P. A., Addis, M. E., Koerner, K., Gollan, J. K., et al. (1996). A component analysis of cognitive-behavioral treatment for depression. *Journal of Consulting and Clinical Psychology, 64*(2), 295–304.

Jahng, K. H., Martin, L. R., Golin, C. E., & DiMatteo, M. R. (2005). Preferences for medical collaboration: Patient–physician congruence and patient outcomes. *Patient Education and Counseling, 57*(3), 308–314.

Janis, I. L., & Mann, L. (1977). *Decision making: A psychological analysis of conflict, choice, and commitment.* New York: Free Press.

Joseph, A. M., Willenbring, M. L., Nugent, S. M., & Nelson, D. B. (2004). A randomized trial of concurrent versus delayed smoking intervention for patients in alcohol dependence treatment. *Journal of Studies on Alcohol, 65*(6), 681–691.

Kaplan, S. H., Greenfield, S., & Ware, J. E., Jr. (1989). Assessing the effects of physician–patient interactions on the outcomes of chronic disease. *Medical Care, 27*(3), S110–S127.

Kavanagh, D. J., Sitharthan, T., Spilsbury, G., & Vignaendra, S. (1999). An evaluation of brief correspondence programs for problem drinkers. *Behavior Therapy, 30*(4), 641–656.

Kazantzis, N., Deane, F. P., & Ronan, K. R. (2000). Homework assignments in cognitive and behavioral therapy: A meta-analysis. *Clinical Psychology: Science and Practice, 7*, 189–202.

Keller, C. S., & McGowan, N. (2001). Examination of the processes of change, decisional balance, self-efficacy for smoking and the stages of change in Mexican American women. *Southern Online Journal of Nursing Research, 2*(4). Retrieved from *www.resourcenter.net/images/snrs/files/sojnr_articles/iss04vol02.htm*.

Kertes, A., Westra, H., & Aviram, A. (2009). *Therapist effects in cognitive behavioral therapy: Client perspectives*. Paper presented at the 117th Annual Convention of the American Psychological Association, Toronto, ON, Canada.

Kiene, S. M., & Barta, W. D. (2006). A brief individualized computer-delivered sexual risk reduction intervention increases HIV/AIDS preventive behavior. *Journal of Adolescent Health, 39*(3), 404–410.

Kiernan, M., Moore, S. D., Schoffman, D. E., Lee, K., King, A. C., Taylor, C. B., et al. (2012). Social support for healthy behaviors: Scale psychometrics and prediction of weight loss among women in a behavioral program. *Obesity, 20*(4), 756–764.

King, A. C., Castro, C. M., Buman, M. P., Hekler, E. B., Urizar Jr., G. G., & Ahn, D. K. (2013). Behavioral impacts of sequentially versus simultaneously delivered dietary plus physical activity interventions: The CALM trial. *Annals of Behavioral Medicine, 46*(2), 157–168.

Kozak, A. T., & Fought, A. (2011). Beyond alcohol and drug addiction: Does the negative trait of low distress tolerance have an association with overeating? *Appetite, 57*(3), 578–581.

Krupnick, J. L., Sotsky, S. M., Simmens, S., Moyer, J., Elkin, I., Watkins, J., et al. (1996). The role of the therapeutic alliance in psychotherapy and pharmacotherapy outcome: Findings in the National Institute of Mental Health Treatment of Depression Collaborative Research Program. *Journal of Consulting and Clinical Psychology, 64*(3), 532–539.

Kurtz, M. M., & Mueser, K. T. (2008). A meta-analysis of controlled research on social skills training for schizophrenia. *Journal of Consulting and Clinical Psychology, 76*(3), 491–504.

Lam, D., & Wong, G. (2005). Prodromes, coping strategies and psychological interventions in bipolar disorders. *Clinical Psychology Review, 25*(8), 1028–1042.

Lambert, M. J., & Barley, D. E. (2001). Research summary on the therapeutic relationship and psychotherapy outcome. *Psychotherapy: Theory, Research, Practice, Training, 38*(4), 357–361.

Leahy, R. L. (2003). *Roadblocks in cognitive-behavioral therapy: Transforming challenges into opportunities for change*. New York: Cambridge University Press.

LeBeau, R. T., Davies, C. D., Culver, N. C., & Craske, M. G. (2013). Homework compliance counts in cognitive-behavioral therapy. *Cognitive Behaviour Therapy,* 42(3), 171–179.

Lepper, M. R., Corpus, J. H., & Iyengar, S. S. (2005). Intrinsic and extrinsic motivational orientations in the classroom: Age differences and academic correlates. *Journal of Educational Psychology,* 97(2), 184–196.

Leyro, T. M., Zvolensky, M. J., & Bernstein, A. (2010). Distress tolerance and psychopathological symptoms and disorders: A review of the empirical literature among adults. *Psychological Bulletin,* 136(4), 576–600.

Linehan, M. M. (1993). *Cognitive-behavioral treatment of borderline personality disorder.* New York: Guilford Press.

Lobban, F., & Barrowclough, C. (Eds.). (2009). *A casebook of family interventions for psychosis.* Chichester, West Sussex, UK: Wiley.

Lorig, K. R., Ritter, P., Stewart, A. L., Sobel, D. S., Brown, B. W., Jr., Bandura, A., et al. (2001). Chronic disease self-management program: 2-year health status and health care utilization outcomes. *Medical Care,* 39(11), 1217–1223.

Luborsky, L., Crits-Christoph, P., Alexander, L., Margolis, M., & Cohen, M. (1983). Two helping alliance methods for predicting outcomes of psychotherapy: A counting signs vs. a global rating method. *Journal of Nervous and Mental Disease,* 171(8), 480–491.

Lundahl, B., & Burke, B. L. (2009). The effectiveness and applicability of motivational interviewing: A practice-friendly review of four meta-analyses. *Journal of Clinical Psychology,* 65(11), 1232–1245.

Lynch, M. F., Vansteenkiste, M., Deci, E. L., & Ryan, R. M. (2011). Autonomy as process and outcome: Revisiting cultural and practical issues in motivation for counseling. *The Counseling Psychologist,* 39, 286–302.

Magill, M., & Ray, L. A. (2009). Cognitive-behavioral treatment with adult alcohol and illicit drug users: A meta-analysis of randomized controlled trials. *Journal of Studies on Alcohol and Drugs,* 70(4), 516–527.

Marcus, B. H., Dubbert, P. M., Forsyth, L. H., McKenzie, T. L., Stone, E. J., Dunn, A. L., et al. (2000). Physical activity behavior change: Issues in adoption and maintenance. *Health Psychology,* 19(1S), 32–41.

Marlatt, G. A., & Donovan, D. M. (2005). *Relapse prevention: Maintenance strategies in the treatment of addictive behaviors* (2nd ed.). New York: Guilford Press.

Marlatt, G. A., & George, W. H. (1984). Relapse prevention: Introduction and overview of the model. *British Journal of Addiction,* 79(3), 261–273.

Marlatt, G. A., & Gordon, J. R. (1985). Relapse prevention: A self-control strategy for the maintenance of behavior change. In G. A. Marlatt & J. R. Gordon (Eds.), *Relapse prevention: Maintenance strategies in the treatment of addictive behaviors* (1st ed., pp. 85–101). New York: Guilford Press.

Martell, C., Dimidjian, S., & Herman-Dunn, R. (2010). *Behavioral activation for depression: A clinician's guide.* New York: Guilford Press.

Mausbach, B. T., Moore, R., Roesch, S., Cardenas, V., & Patterson, T. L. (2010). The relationship between homework compliance and therapy outcomes: An updated meta-analysis. *Cognitive Therapy and Research,* 34(5), 429–438.

Mazzucchelli, T., Kane, R., & Rees, C. (2009). Behavioral activation treatments for depression in adults: A meta-analysis and review. *Clinical Psychology: Science and Practice, 16*(4), 383–411.

McEvoy, P. M., Nathan, P., & Norton, P. J. (2009). Efficacy of transdiagnostic treatments: A review of published outcome studies and future research directions. *Journal of Cognitive Psychotherapy, 23*(1), 20–33.

McGowan, S. K., & Behar, E. (2013). A preliminary investigation of stimulus control training for worry: Effects on anxiety and insomnia. *Behavior Modification, 37*(1), 90–112.

McHugh, R. K., Hearon, B. A., & Otto, M. W. (2010). Cognitive behavioral therapy for substance use disorders. *Psychiatric Clinics of North America, 33*(3), 511–525.

McHugh, R. K., Murray, H. W., & Barlow, D. H. (2009). Balancing fidelity and adaptation in the dissemination of empirically-supported treatments: The promise of trans-diagnostic interventions. *Behaviour Research and Therapy, 47*(11), 946–953.

McIntosh, B., Yu, C., Lal, A., Chelak, K., Cameron, C., Singh, S., et al. (2010). Efficacy of self-monitoring of blood glucose in patients with type 2 diabetes mellitus managed without insulin: A systematic review and meta-analysis. *Open Medicine, 4*(2), 102–113.

McKay, J. R., Alterman, A. I., Cacciola, J. S., O'Brien, C. P., Koppenhaver, J. M., & Shepard, D. S. (1999). Continuing care for cocaine dependence: Comprehensive 2-year outcomes. *Journal of Consulting and Clinical Psychology, 67*(3), 420–427.

McKee, S. A., Carroll, K. M., Sinha, R., Robinson, J. E., Nich, C., Cavallo, D., et al. (2007). Enhancing brief cognitive-behavioral therapy with motivational enhancement techniques in cocaine users. *Drug and Alcohol Dependence, 91*(1), 97–101.

Miller, W. R. (1999). *Integrating spirituality into treatment: Resources for practitioners.* Washington, DC: American Psychological Association.

Miller, W. R. (2004). *Combined behavioral intervention manual: A clinical research guide for therapists treating people with alcohol abuse and dependence* (Vol. 1). Bethesda, MD: National Institute on Alcohol Abuse and Alcoholism.

Miller, W. R. (2012). MI and psychotherapy. *Motivational Interviewing: Training, Research, Implementation, Practice, 1*(1), 2–6.

Miller, W. R., Forcehimes, A. A., & Zweben, A. (2011). *Treating addiction: A guide for professionals.* New York: Guilford Press.

Miller, W. R., & Hester, R. K. (1986). The effectiveness of alcoholism treatment. In W. R. Miller & N. Heather (Eds.), *Treating addictive behaviors: Processes of change* (pp. 121–174). New York: Springer.

Miller, W. R., & Moyers, T. B. (2015). The forest and the trees: Relational and specific factors in addiction treatment. *Addiction, 110*(3), 401–413.

Miller, W. R., Moyers, T. B., Arciniega, L., Ernst, D., & Forcehimes, A. (2005, July). Training, supervision and quality monitoring of the COMBINE Study behavioral interventions. *Journal of Studies on Alcohol* (Suppl. 15), 188–195.

Miller, W. R., & Rollnick, S. (Eds.). (2002). *Motivational interviewing: Preparing people for change* (2nd ed.). New York: Guilford Press.

Miller, W. R., & Rollnick, S. (2009). Ten things that motivational interviewing is not. *Behavioural and Cognitive Psychotherapy, 37*(02), 129–140.

Miller, W. R., & Rollnick, S. (2012). *Motivational interviewing: Helping people change* (3rd ed.). New York: Guilford Press.

Miller, W. R., Taylor, C. A., & West, J. C. (1980). Focused versus broad-spectrum behavior therapy for problem drinkers. *Journal of Consulting and Clinical Psychology, 48*(5), 590–601.

Miller, W. R., Zweben, A., & DiClemente, C. C. (1994). *Motivational enhancement therapy manual* (Project Match Monograph Series, Vol. 2). Washington, DC: National Institute on Alcohol Abuse and Alcoholism.

Milroy, L., & Muysken, P. (1995). *One speaker, two languages: Cross-disciplinary perspectives on code-switching.* Cambridge, UK: Cambridge University Press.

Miltenberger, R. (2008). Behavioral skills training procedures. In *Behaviour modification: Principles and procedures* (pp. 251–265). Belmont, CA: Thomson.

Minami, T., Wampold, B. E., Serlin, R. C., Hamilton, E. G., Brown, G. S. J., & Kircher, J. C. (2008). Benchmarking the effectiveness of psychotherapy treatment for adult depression in a managed care environment: A preliminary study. *Journal of Consulting and Clinical Psychology, 76*(1), 116–124.

Monti, P. M., & O'Leary, T. A. (1999). Coping and social skills training for alcohol and cocaine dependence. *Psychiatric Clinics of North America, 22*(2), 447–470.

Moulds, M. L., & Nixon, R. D. (2006). *In vivo* flooding for anxiety disorders: Proposing its utility in the treatment of posttraumatic stress disorder. *Journal of Anxiety Disorders, 20*(4), 498–509.

Moyers, T. B., & Houck, J. (2011). Combining motivational interviewing with cognitive-behavioral treatments for substance abuse: Lessons from the COMBINE research project. *Cognitive and Behavioral Practice, 18*(1), 38–45.

Moyers, T., Martin, T., Catley, D., Harris, K. J., & Ahluwalia, J. S. (2003). Assessing the integrity of motivational interviewing: Reliability of the motivational interviewing skills code. *Behavioural and Cognitive Psychotherapy, 31*(2), 177–184.

Moyers, T. B., Martin, T., Christopher, P. J., Houck, J. M., Tonigan, J. S., & Amrhein, P. C. (2007). Client language as a mediator of motivational interviewing efficacy: Where is the evidence? *Alcoholism: Clinical and Experimental Research, 31*(10, Suppl.), 40S–47S.

Moyers, T. B., Martin, T., Manuel, J. K., Hendrickson, S. M. L., & Miller, W. R. (2005). Assessing competence in the use of motivational interviewing. *Journal of Substance Abuse Treatment, 28*(1), 19–26.

Mueser, K. T., & Drake, R. E. (2007). Comorbidity: What have we learned and where are we going? *Clinical Psychology: Science and Practice, 14*(1), 64–69.

Naar, S., & Flynn, H. (2015). Client language as a mediator of motivational interviewing efficacy: Where is the evidence? In H. Arkowitz, W. R. Miller, & S. Rollnick (Eds.), *Motivational interviewing in the treatment of psychological problems* (2nd ed., pp. 170–192). New York: Guilford Press.

Naar-King, S., Earnshaw, P., & Breckon, J. (2013). Toward a universal maintenance intervention: Integrating cognitive-behavioral treatment with motivational interviewing for maintenance of behavior change. *Journal of Cognitive Psychotherapy, 27*(2), 126–137.

Naar-King, S., Ellis, D. A., Idalski Carcone, A., Templin, T., Jacques-Tiura, A. J., Brogan Hartlieb, K., et al. (2016). Sequential Multiple Assignment Randomized Trial (SMART) to construct weight loss interventions for African American adolescents. *Journal of Clinical Child and Adolescent Psychology, 45*(4), 428–441.

Naar-King, S., Outlaw, A. Y., Sarr, M., Parsons, J. T., Belzer, M., Macdonell, K., et al. (2013). Motivational Enhancement System for Adherence (MESA): Pilot randomized trial of a brief computer-delivered prevention intervention for youth initiating antiretroviral treatment. *Journal of Pediatric Psychology, 38*(6), 638–648.

Newman, M., & Borkovec, T. (1995). Cognitive-behavioral treatment of generalized anxiety disorder. *The Clinical Psychologist, 48*(4), 5–7.

Newman, M. G., Consoli, A. J., & Taylor, C. B. (1999). A palmtop computer program for the treatment of generalized anxiety disorder. *Behavior Modification, 23*(4), 597–619.

Nickoletti, P., & Taussig, H. N. (2006). Outcome expectancies and risk behaviors in maltreated adolescents. *Journal of Research on Adolescence, 16*(2), 217–228.

Nigg, C. R., Borrelli, B., Maddock, J., & Dishman, R. K. (2008). A theory of physical activity maintenance. *Applied Psychology, 57*(4), 544–560.

Nock, M., & Kazdin, A. E. (2005). Randomized controlled trial of a brief intervention for increasing participation in parent management training. *Journal of Consulting and Clinical Psychology, 73*(5), 872–879.

Norton, P. J. (2012). A randomized clinical trial of transdiagnostic cognitive-behavioral treatments for anxiety disorder by comparison to relaxation training. *Behavior Therapy, 43*(3), 506–517.

O'Connell, K. A., Cook, M. R., Gerkovich, M. M., Potocky, M., & Swan, G. E. (1990). Reversal theory and smoking: A state-based approach to ex-smokers' highly tempting situations. *Journal of Consulting and Clinical Psychology, 58*(4), 489–494.

Olander, E. K., Fletcher, H., Williams, S., Atkinson, L., Turner, A., & French, D. P. (2013). What are the most effective techniques in changing obese individuals' physical activity self-efficacy and behaviour: A systematic review and meta-analysis. *International Journal of Behavioral Nutrition and Physical Activity, 10*, 29.

Ondersma, S. J., Chase, S. K., Svikis, D., & Schuster, C. R. (2005). Computer-based brief motivational intervention for perinatal drug use. *Journal of Substance Abuse Treatment, 28*(4), 305–312.

Ondersma, S. J., Svikis, D. S., Lam, P. K., Connors-Burge, V. S., Ledgerwood, D. M., & Hopper, J. A. (2012). A randomized trial of computer-delivered brief intervention and low-intensity contingency management for smoking during pregnancy. *Nicotine and Tobacco Research, 14*(3), 351–360.

Ondersma, S. J., Svikis, D. S., & Schuster, C. R. (2007). Computer-based brief intervention: A randomized trial with postpartum women. *American Journal of Preventive Medicine, 32*(3), 231–238.

Ondersma, S. J., Svikis, D. S., Thacker, L. R., Beatty, J. R., & Lockhart, N. (2014). Computer-delivered screening and brief intervention (e-SBI) for postpartum drug use: A randomized trial. *Journal of Substance Abuse Treatment, 46*(1), 52–59.

Ong, L. M., De Haes, J. C., Hoos, A. M., & Lammes, F. B. (1995). Doctor–patient communication: A review of the literature. *Social Science and Medicine, 40*(7), 903–918.

Orsega-Smith, E. M., Payne, L. L., Mowen, A. J., Ho, C.-H., & Godbey, G. C. (2007). The role of social support and self-efficacy in shaping the leisure time physical activity of older adults. *Journal of Leisure Research, 39*(4), 705–727.

Oser, M. L., Trafton, J. A., Lejuez, C. W., & Bonn-Miller, M. O. (2013). Differential associations between perceived and objective measurement of distress tolerance in relation to antiretroviral treatment adherence and response among HIV-positive individuals. *Behavior Therapy, 44*(3), 432–442.

Osilla, K. C., Hepner, K. A., Muñoz, R. F., Woo, S., & Watkins, K. (2009). Developing an integrated treatment for substance use and depression using cognitive-behavioral therapy. *Journal of Substance Abuse Treatment, 37*(4), 412–420.

Öst, L.-G., Alm, T., Brandberg, M., & Breitholtz, E. (2001). One vs five sessions of exposure and five sessions of cognitive therapy in the treatment of claustrophobia. *Behaviour Research and Therapy, 39*(2), 167–183.

Ougrin, D. (2011). Efficacy of exposure versus cognitive therapy in anxiety disorders: Systematic review and meta-analysis. *BMC Psychiatry, 11*(1), 1.

Padesky, C. A. (1993). *Socratic questioning: Changing minds or guiding discovery.* Keynote address delivered at the European Congress of Behavioural and Cognitive Therapies, London.

Papworth, M., Marrinan, T., Martin, B., Keegan, D., & Chaddock, A. (2013). *Low intensity cognitive-behaviour therapy: A practitioner's guide.* London: SAGE.

Parsons, J. T., Golub, S. A., Rosof, E., & Holder, C. (2007). Motivational interviewing and cognitive-behavioral intervention to improve HIV medication adherence among hazardous drinkers: A randomized controlled trial. *Journal of Acquired Immune Deficiency Syndrome, 46*(4), 443–450.

Paul, R., & Elder, L. (2006). *Thinker's guide to the art of Socratic questioning.* Tomales, CA: Foundation for Critical Thinking.

Perri, M. G., Sears, S. F., & Clark, J. E. (1993). Strategies for improving maintenance of weight loss: Toward a continuous care model of obesity management. *Diabetes Care, 16*(1), 200–209.

Piasecki, T. M. (2006). Relapse to smoking. *Clinical Psychology Review, 26*(2), 196–215.

Polivy, J., & Herman, C. P. (2002). If at first you don't succeed: False hopes of self-change. *The American Psychologist, 57*(9), 677–689.

Powers, M. B., & Emmelkamp, P. M. (2008). Virtual reality exposure therapy for anxiety disorders: A meta-analysis. *Journal of Anxiety Disorders, 22*(3), 561–569.

Prochaska, J. J., & Prochaska, J. O. (2011). A review of multiple health behavior change interventions for primary prevention. *American Journal of Lifestyle Medicine, 5*(3), 208–221.

Prochaska, J. J., Spring, B., & Nigg, C. R. (2008). Multiple health behavior change research: An introduction and overview. *Preventive Medicine, 46*(3), 181–188.

Prochaska, J. O., Velicer, W. F., Rossi, J. S., Goldstein, M. G., Marcus, B. H., Rakowski, W., et al. (1994). Stages of change and decisional balance for 12 problem behaviors. *Health Psychology, 13*(1), 39–46.

Resnicow, K., & McMaster, F. (2012). Motivational interviewing: Moving from why to how with autonomy support. *International Journal of Behavioral Nutrition and Physical Activity, 9*(1), 1.

Resnicow, K., McMaster, F., & Rollnick, S. (2012). Action reflections: A client-centered technique to bridge the WHY–HOW transition in motivational interviewing. *Behavioural and Cognitive Psychotherapy, 40*(4), 474–480.

Ries, R. (1996). *Assessment and treatment of patients with coexisting mental illness and alcohol and other drug abuse.* Darby, PA: Diane.

Riper, H., Andersson, G., Hunter, S. B., Wit, J., Berking, M., & Cuijpers, P. (2014). Treatment of comorbid alcohol use disorders and depression with cognitive-behavioural therapy and motivational interviewing: A meta-analysis. *Addiction, 109*(3), 394–406.

Rogers, C. (1951). *Client-centered therapy: Its current practice, implications and theory.* London: Constable.

Rollnick, S., Miller, W. R., & Butler, C. C. (2008). *Motivational interviewing in health care: Helping patients change behavior.* New York: Guilford Press.

Rosengren, D. B. (2009). *Building motivational interviewing skills: A practitioner workbook.* New York: Guilford Press.

Safren, S. A., Otto, M. W., Worth, J. L., Salomon, E., Johnson, W., Mayer, K., et al. (2001). Two strategies to increase adherence to HIV antiretroviral medication: Life-steps and medication monitoring. *Behaviour Research and Therapy, 39*(10), 1151–1162.

Safren, S., Perlman, C., Sprich, S., & Otto, M. (2005). *Mastering your adult ADHD: A cognitive behavioral treatment program—Therapist guide.* New York: Oxford University Press.

Schwartz, R. P., Gryczynski, J., Mitchell, S. G., Gonzales, A., Moseley, A., Peterson, T. R., et al. (2014). Computerized versus in-person brief intervention for drug misuse: A randomized clinical trial. *Addiction, 109*(7), 1091–1098.

Smith, D. E., Heckemeyer, C. M., Kratt, P. P., & Mason, D. A. (1997). Motivational interviewing to improve adherence to a behavioral weight-control program for older obsese women with NIDDM. *Diabetes Care, 20*(1), 52–54.

Sobell, M. B., Bogardis, J., Schuller, R., Leo, G. I., & Sobell, L. C. (1989). Is self-monitoring of alcohol consumption reactive? *Behavioral Assessment, 11*(4), 447–458.

Spoelstra, S. L., Schueller, M., Hilton, M., & Ridenour, K. (2015). Interventions combining motivational interviewing and cognitive behaviour to promote medication adherence: A literature review. *Journal of Clinical Nursing, 24*(9–10), 1163–1173.

Spring, B., Doran, N., Pagoto, S., Schneider, K., Pingitore, R., & Hedeker, D. (2004). Randomized controlled trial for behavioral smoking and weight control treatment: Effect of concurrent versus sequential intervention. *Journal of Consulting and Clinical Psychology, 72*(5), 785–796.

Stetler, C. B., Damschroder, L. J., Helfrich, C. D., & Hagedorn, H. J. (2011). A guide for applying a revised version of the PARIHS framework for implementation. *Implementation Science, 6*(1), 99.

Stewart, M., Brown, J., Donner, A., McWhinney, I., Oates, J., Weston, W., et al. (2000). The impact of patient-centered care on outcomes. *Journal of Family Practice, 49*(9), 796–804.

Stotts, A. L., Schmitz, J. M., Rhoades, H. M., & Grabowski, J. (2001). Motivational interviewing with cocaine-dependent patients: A pilot study. *Journal of Consulting and Clinical Psychology, 69*(5), 858–862.

Street, R. L., Jr., Gordon, H., & Haidet, P. (2007). Physicians' communication and perceptions of patients: Is it how they look, how they talk, or is it just the doctor? *Social Science and Medicine, 65*(3), 586–598.

Strickler, D. C. (2011). Requiring case management meetings to be conducted outside the clinic. *Psychiatric Services, 62*(10), 1215–1217.

Sturmey, P. (2009). Behavioral activation is an evidence-based treatment for depression. *Behavior Modification, 33*(6), 818–829.

Surgeon General. (1999). *Mental health: A report of the Surgeon General.* Bethesda, MD: U.S. Public Health Service.

Sweet, S. N., & Fortier, M. S. (2010). Improving physical activity and dietary behaviours with single or multiple health behaviour interventions?: A synthesis of meta-analyses and reviews. *International Journal of Environmental Research and Public Health, 7*(4), 1720–1743.

Tolin, D. F. (2010). Is cognitive-behavioral therapy more effective than other therapies?: A meta-analytic review. *Clinical Psychology Review, 30*(6), 710–720.

Trummer, U. F., Mueller, U. O., Nowak, P., Stidl, T., & Pelikan, J. M. (2006). Does physician–patient communication that aims at empowering patients improve clinical outcome?: A case study. *Patient Education and Counseling, 61*(2), 299–306.

Turner, J. S., & Leach, D. J. (2009). Brief behavioural activation treatment of chronic anxiety in an older adult. *Behaviour Change, 26*(3), 214–222.

Tzilos, G. K., Sokol, R. J., & Ondersma, S. J. (2011). A randomized phase I trial of a brief computer-delivered intervention for alcohol use during pregnancy. *Journal of Women's Health, 20*(10), 1517–1524.

Uhlig, K., Patel, K., Ip, S., Kitsios, G. D., & Balk, E. M. (2013). Self-measured blood pressure monitoring in the management of hypertension: A systematic review and meta-analysis. *Annals of Internal Medicine, 159*(3), 185–194.

Utay, J., & Miller, M. (2006). Guided imagery as an effective therapeutic technique: A brief review of its history and efficacy research. *Journal of Instructional Psychology, 33*(1), 40–44.

Valle, S. K. (1981). Interpersonal functioning of alcoholism counselors and treatment outcome. *Journal of Studies on Alcohol, 42*(9), 783–790.

Vallerand, R. J. (1997). Toward a hierarchical model of intrinsic and extrinsic motivation. *Advances in Experimental Social Psychology, 29*, 271–360.

Vandelanotte, C., De Bourdeaudhuij, I., Sallis, J. F., Spittaels, H., & Brug, J. (2005). Efficacy of sequential or simultaneous interactive computer-tailored interventions for increasing physical activity and decreasing fat intake. *Annals of Behavioral Medicine, 29*(2), 138–146.

Verkuil, B., Brosschot, J. F., Korrelboom, K., Reul-Verlaan, R., & Thayer, J. F. (2011). Pretreatment of worry enhances the effects of stress management therapy: A randomized clinical trial. *Psychotherapy and Psychosomatics, 80*(3), 189–190.

Vincze, G., Barner, J. C., & Lopez, D. (2003). Factors associated with adherence to self-monitoring of blood glucose among persons with diabetes. *The Diabetes Educator, 30*(1), 112–125.

Walters, G. D. (2001). Behavioral self-control training for problem drinkers: A meta-analysis of randomized control studies. *Behavior Therapy, 31*(1), 135–149.

Walters, S. T., Vader, A. M., Harris, T. R., Field, C. A., & Jouriles, E. N. (2009). Dismantling motivational interviewing and feedback for college drinkers: A randomized clinical trial. *Journal of Consulting and Clinical Psychology, 77*(1), 64–73.

Weiss, C. V., Mills, J. S., Westra, H. A., & Carter, J. C. (2013). A preliminary study of motivational interviewing as a prelude to intensive treatment for an eating disorder. *Journal of Eating Disorders, 1*(1), 1.

Westmaas, J. L., Bontemps-Jones, J., & Bauer, J. E. (2010). Social support in smoking cessation: Reconciling theory and evidence. *Nicotine and Tobacco Research, 12*(7), 695–707.

Westra, H. A., & Arkowitz, H. (2011). Introduction. *Cognitive and Behavioral Practice, 18*(1), 1–4.

Westra, H. A., Arkowitz, H., & Dozois, D. J. (2009). Adding a motivational interviewing pretreatment to cognitive behavioral therapy for generalized anxiety disorder: A preliminary randomized controlled trial. *Journal of Anxiety Disorders, 23*(8), 1106–1117.

Westra, H. A., Constantino, M. J., Arkowitz, H., & Dozois, D. J. (2011). Therapist differences in cognitive-behavioral psychotherapy for generalized anxiety disorder: A pilot study. *Psychotherapy, 48*(3), 283–292.

Westra, H. A., & Dozois, D. J. (2006). Preparing clients for cognitive behavioral therapy: A randomized pilot study of motivational interviewing for anxiety. *Cognitive Therapy and Research, 30*(4), 481–498.

Wilson, G. T., & Vitousek, K. M. (1999). Self-monitoring in the assessment of eating disorders. *Psychological Assessment, 11*(4), 480–489.

Wing, R. R., & Phelan, S. (2005). Long-term weight loss maintenance. *American Journal of Clinical Nutrition, 82*(1), 222S–225S.

Witkiewitz, K., Lustyk, M. K. B., & Bowen, S. (2013). Re-training the addicted brain: A review of hypothesized neurobiological mechanisms of mindfulness-based relapse prevention. *Psychology of Addictive Behaviors, 27*(2), 351–365.

Witkiewitz, K. A., & Marlatt, G. A. (Eds.). (2007). *Therapist's guide to evidence-based relapse prevention.* Burlington, MA: Elsevier.

Yovel, I., & Safren, S. A. (2007). Measuring homework utility in psychotherapy: Cognitive-behavioral therapy for adult attention-deficit hyperactivity disorder as an example. *Cognitive Therapy and Research, 31*(3), 385–399.

Zvolensky, M. J., Vujanovic, A. A., Bernstein, A., & Leyro, T. (2010). Distress tolerance theory, measurement, and relations to psychopathology. *Current Directions in Psychological Science, 19*(6), 406–410.

Index

Note. "f " or "t" following a page number indicates a figure or a table.

235

Substance use and abuse, 4–5
Suggestions, 43–44, 188. *See also* "Ask–tell–ask" sequence (ATA)
Summarizing. *See also* Reflection
   collaborative assessment and, 39–40
   evaluation and, 44–45, 46*f*
   feedback and, 48*t*
   maintenance and, 187
   overview, 7
   session attendance and, 175
   Socratic questioning and, 115
   training in MI-CBT integration and, 213*t*
   treatment planning and, 52
Sustain talk
   cognitive restructuring and, 111–112
   engagement and, 17–18
   evaluation and, 47
   self-monitoring and, 78–79
   skills training and, 142
   training in MI-CBT integration and, 213*t*
Synthesizing questions, 115–116. *See also* Questions

T

Tasks of treatment, 14–15
Technology, 217
Termination, 194–195, 194*f*. *See also* Maintenance
Therapeutic alliance. *See also* Working alliance
   engagement and, 7, 12–18
   evaluation and, 36
   integrating MI with CBT during the initial sessions and, 29
   overview, 1, 11–12
   self-monitoring and, 79
Thinking errors. *See* Unhelpful thoughts
Thought records, 112–113
Thoughts, 36, 187. *See also* Cognitive restructuring
Time sampling procedures, 80. *See also* Self-monitoring
Tracking. *See* Self-monitoring

Transdiagnostic treatments, 1–2, 5, 9, 202. *See also* Integrated treatment manual
Treatment goals. *See* Goals of treatment
Treatment planning. *See also* Planning
   activities regarding, 56–66
   collaborative assessment and, 39–42, 41*t*
   engagement and, 36–42, 41*t*
   handouts regarding, 67–72
   overview, 35–36, 49–54, 51*f*, 53*f*
   summarizing and, 44–45, 46*f*
Triggers. *See also* Antecedents
   collaborative assessment and, 39–40
   engagement and, 74
   maintenance and, 187–188
   problem-solving skills and, 132
   self-monitoring and, 73–74, 85
Typical Day Exercise, 40, 42

U

Uncertainty, 188–189
Understanding, 15–17, 76*t*
Unhelpful thoughts, 111–112. *See also* Cognitive restructuring
Unified treatments, 1–2

V

Verbal rehearsal, 141
Visualization, 86, 102–103

W

When–then plan, 85. *See also* Planning
Working alliance, 7. *See also* Therapeutic alliance
Worry
   handouts regarding, 161
   self-monitoring and, 79
   stimulus control of, 135–136